Belinda Hollyer has had migr⟨...⟩ ⟨...⟩ ⟨...⟩ ⟨she⟩ learned to spell them, but now (with fingers crossed) thinks she has finally conquered them.

A writer and publishing consultant for the past four years, she has previously worked as a publisher, and a teacher. She has lived in New Zealand, Australia and the Lebanon, and now lives in north London, although she would much rather be on a houseboat in Key West.

Jacky Fleming is a best-selling cartoonist. Her books, *Be a Bloody Train Driver*, *Never Give Up* and *Falling in Love* are published by Penguin.

Also by Belinda Hollyer

Staying Together: Secrets of a Successful Relationship
(Piccadilly Press)

MIND OVER MIGRAINE

The complete
self-help
plan

Belinda Hollyer

HEADLINE

First published in 1994
by HEADLINE BOOK PUBLISHING

10 9 8 7 6 5 4 3 2 1

ISBN 0 7472 4477 4

Typeset by
Letterpart Limited, Reigate, Surrey

Printed and bound in Great Britain by
HarperCollins Manufacturing, Glasgow

HEADLINE BOOK PUBLISHING
A division of Hodder Headline PLC
338 Euston Road
London NW1 3BH

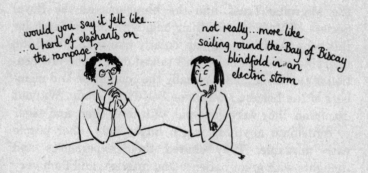

Acknowledgements

I should like to thank the British Migraine Association, the Migraine Trust, and the librarians at the Royal Society of Medicine, for their help with the research for this book. And I should particularly like to thank all the migraine sufferers to whom I talked during the preparation of this book, and especially the committee and members of the Leicester Migraine Self-Help Group. Without exception, they were generous with their time, and eager to contribute anything which might help other people with migraine. They shared their experiences and thoughts with great patience and interest, and I am very grateful to them.

Contents

CHAPTER 1

The Meaning of Migraine

THE WORST HEADACHE IN THE WORLD

If you are reading this book, it's likely that you have experienced at least one migraine headache – or maybe you think you have, but you want to find out for certain. If migraine is a constant problem in your life, you will be expecting help in learning to understand and to manage its effects. Or perhaps you know someone who has migraine, and you want to understand what that means. You are probably looking for facts: about the experience itself; about the symptoms; and about dealing with all of this.

The aim of this book is not only to outline the facts about migraine, but also to provide real help in tackling it. The symptoms of migraine *can* be alleviated, controlled, and even entirely avoided. You *can* help yourself towards a migraine-free existence, and others can help you along the road.

It takes patience, careful planning, and a persistent sort of stubbornness to challenge migraine; it also takes time. And the first step towards success is to learn as much as you can about the enemy: this thing called migraine. What is it?

1

GETTING YOUR HEAD ROUND THE FACTS

A lot of misunderstandings, misconceptions, and plain untruths surround the whole area of migraine. Scientists and doctors find it a difficult subject to get to grips with, because the main symptom of migraine – the headache – is a subjective one.

A rash, for example, can be observed by an outsider. It can be compared with other rashes. It could even be measured on a scale in a laboratory. But a headache can only be described by the sufferer. One migraine expert has said that studying migraine is rather like trying to study the force of gravity – you can only observe its effects!

Don't lose your head

Another problem is that migraine seems to involve a bewildering range of factors. The list of possible triggers that can set off a migraine is extremely long, and the possible accompanying symptoms range very widely. More confusing still, neither the triggers nor the symptoms are necessarily consistent, even for one sufferer. Your migraine may begin with a certain set of symptoms when you are in your teens or twenties, say – but ten years later, the symptoms may have altered quite dramatically. And what triggers your migraine one week – drinking red wine, for instance – may have no effect whatsoever at another time. This makes migraine hard to define, as well as difficult to treat.

So I want to start with some certainties, by clearing away some of the popular misconceptions about migraine, and by establishing what *isn't* true and what *may* be true – as well as what is known for sure.

MORE THAN A HEADACHE

A migraine is not just an ordinary headache with a fancy name. It isn't life-threatening, although it can certainly *feel* as bad as that when you're having a migraine attack. But the pain is not a symptom of anything more serious; migraine is not a malignant condition. Other sorts of headache can sometimes be a warning of a serious medical problem but a migraine headache is not that sort of symptom. And although migraine is medically recognised, and although lots of money and effort has been spent on migraine research, its precise causes are still unknown.

Migraine is a pattern of symptoms which together form a medical condition; the headache (which is often what people mean when they say they have a migraine) is just a part of the pattern, one of the symptoms of the whole condition.

Migraine does not relate to a problem in the structure of your body; it doesn't suggest the hidden existence of a tumour or an abscess, or any other abnormality or peculiarity of that sort. Migraine relates to the way the systems of your body function, and to how they react to certain sets of circumstances. But no one knows exactly what the circumstances are which cause migraine, and so no one yet knows how to cure it.

NOBODY KNOWS EXCEPT YOU

Migraine has an unusually wide range of possible symptoms. If you do suffer from it, your symptoms probably won't be exactly the same as those of another migraine sufferer, and they might even be markedly different. Your own experience of migraine may vary from one attack to the next, and from one stage of your life to another.

The only reliably common factor is the intermittent headache itself, which usually (but not always) occurs on one side of the head. The pain is often intense, but migraine sufferers are also completely free from headaches between attacks. A constant, 'permanent' headache is not a migraine.

No one who has *not* had a migraine can ever truly understand what it's like. It isn't just a bad headache – at its worst it is a debilitating and distressing condition that can send the sufferer to bed for hours, or even days on end. The associated symptoms can include nausea and vomiting, a loss of part of the vision in one or both eyes, a numbness in arms or face or both, giddiness and disturbances in balance, changes in appetite and mood, digestive upsets, and a violent intolerance of certain smells, noises, or tastes.

LIVING WITH MIGRAINE

If you're lucky, your symptoms are only mild ones, and you may be able to function more or less normally whilst you are in the grips of a migraine attack. But others are not so fortunate.

Many sufferers are crippled by the pain, and made helpless by the attendant symptoms. They dread the next attack; they make elaborate efforts to avoid it; their social and personal lives are haunted by the fear of it. Many have lost their jobs, or have been forced to seek alternative employment. Others find that family life inevitably becomes focused exclusively on the needs of the migraine sufferer, which often leads to more anxiety, and to understandable resentments from other family members. Migraine can be a very destructive force, and many people suffer alone, in isolation and misery. Very often, family, friends, employers, and – it has to be said – even doctors, don't understand.

Betty is forty-one, and has had acute attacks of migraine since she was twenty-six. 'I never go out with my family,' she said. 'I'm too frightened that I'll get a migraine, and then the whole evening will be ruined for the family as well as me. If we went out to dinner, a smoker at the next table could start me up. So can some food additives. Sometimes bright light can bring it on, so I have to avoid the cinema. I feel dreadful about it, as though I'm less human than other people.'

'I feel bitterly resentful about the time it's stolen from my life,' another woman told me. 'Once, when I felt very depressed about the frequency of my migraine attacks, I worked out that I'd spent about twelve years of my life vomiting in the dark, in dreadful pain. Then I sat and cried about the way in which migraine was ruining my life. And *then* I decided I had to find out how to stop it!'

You're not alone
From the most recent evidence, it is clear that about 10% of the world's population suffer from migraine at some time in their lives. That figure, however, is estimated from the number of patients whose condition has been reported to – and diagnosed by – doctors, and so it is based on those people whose migraines are bad enough, regular enough, and persistent enough to make them seek medical help. Many more people whose

attacks are mild or infrequent, whose condition has not been diagnosed, or whose symptoms do not fit the current definitions of migraine, are excluded from the estimate. So the true percentage may well be close to 15%, or even higher. Recent studies suggest that 8% of men, and 25% of women, experience migraine at some stage of their lives.

There's a lot of it about

Migraine statistics are calculated from evidence which has been gathered almost exclusively in the western world, but it is highly unlikely that migraine is simply a western phenomenon, or that its causes can be directly related to any of the problems which bedevil the industrialised world. Migraine has been around for too long for that to be a sensible argument.

Even prehistoric peoples may have known about migraine, and tried to cure it. Archaeologists have discovered evidence of trepanned skulls amongst the human remains of neolithic and bronze age times. (Trepanning involves cutting away a section of bone from the skull to leave a small permanent hole.) In these cases, trepanning may well have been a treatment to allow 'evil spirits' to escape, for such methods have been recorded amongst tribal peoples, even in modern times. Perhaps trepanning was a primitive attempt to cure migrainous headaches – a somewhat drastic form of radical surgery going back ten thousand years.

(And just in case you're tempted to feel smug about how far modern medical science has taken us away from such primitive remedies – don't! Horrifyingly, various forms of surgery are still sometimes recommended today for migraine, despite a complete lack of evidence that surgery will help. If it's suggested to you, change your doctor.)

The first written description of migraine attacks so far discovered is more than three and a half thousand years old: an Egyptian papyrus written about 1700 BC mentions an illness of 'half the head'. The Greek physician Galen, who lived from AD 130 to 200, introduced the term 'hemicrania' – or 'half-head' – and it is from later modifications of that word, such as 'megrim', that our present term 'migraine' comes. (That historical link is also the reason why some people insist that pronouncing it as 'me-grain' rather than 'my-grain', is correct. In general, the British tend to say 'me-grain', while Americans and Australians tend to say 'my-grain'. On the other hand, Dr Oliver Sacks, the great migraine authority, says 'my-grain', so you might as well please yourself.)

There are many famous historical examples of migraine. Hippocrates described them; Julius Caesar had them; and in more recent times Mary Tudor, Peter the Great, Charles Darwin, George Eliot, Lewis Carroll, and Sigmund Freud all apparently suffered from them. At least, you may think, you are in interesting company.

SUPERIOR BEINGS?

At one time it was thought that having migraines was a sign of high intelligence – which may *possibly* have been some sort of grim comfort for the sufferers, but in any case is unlikely to be true: it's not just in the mind, and it's not all in the brain, either! No survey has ever shown a correlation between having migraines and scoring well on intelligence tests, nor indeed that there is any significant difference between the intelligence scores of people with, and without, experience of migraines. The idea probably arose through association with all the famous names; even perhaps as an attempt to create a positive aspect which sufferers could share – a sort of consolation prize. ('Oh, what a price I have to pay for my sensitive and highly strung intelligence!')

On the other hand, it may *well* be true that those who consult doctors about their migraines, and who attempt to find ways to control or cure the condition, are of necessity persistent, highly motivated, and very determined – but that's another matter!

Are you the type?

The idea that people who get migraines tend to have a certain sort of personality has been around for as long as the 'high intelligence' claim. Migraineurs – the term for those who suffer from migraine – are said to be typically hard-working, conscientious perfectionists. They easily become anxious in response to stress, and they tend to be both rigid and ambitious. They may also be especially likely to suffer from depression.

There is no reliable scientific evidence to support any of that, but it is interesting that at least some aspects of the migraine personality idea are still used by some researchers dealing with patients who attend migraine clinics, and amongst those doctors who take a close interest in the subject.

According to one recent report, migraineurs score highly on two particular areas of personality. They feel especially guilty if things for which they are responsible are not well done, or have to be left incomplete; they also tend to take criticism very much to heart. And secondly, although they may seem outwardly calm and collected, they do not easily tolerate frustration, or deal with it in a constructive way.

Could all this be true? And even if it is true, is it a cause, or a result? Is this yet another version of the old chicken-and-egg problem: which comes first, the migraine or the depression? Does the migraine syndrome create circumstances in which people feel especially guilty, and feel responsible for more than their fair share of problems?

Certainly, relaxation techniques, self-hypnosis, and other related forms of self-help therapy discussed later in this book should be especially useful forms of treatment to try if you think the description fits you. Turning 'I can't relax!' into 'I'll learn *how* to relax!' is the key to success for many people.

But you should also guard against accepting the notion of a 'migraine personality' too readily. This can easily lead to the view that having a migraine attack is, in some way, the 'fault' of the migraineur. There is no justice in a migraine attack. It is not the result of 'doing something wrong', and in fact the very characteristics which are attributed to migraineurs are ones which our society generally values and admires! Migraineurs have enough problems without taking the blame for their symptoms as well as having to suffer them.

RELATIVELY SPEAKING

Migraine usually runs in families. If you have migraines, there is a more than 60% chance that you have a close relative who also gets migraine. So prevalent is the family connection, in fact, that having another sufferer in your family was once one of the medical criteria used to diagnose migraine.

Keeping it in the family

The family factor doesn't necessarily mean that migraine is an inherited condition, of course. It could be a copied response to certain situations, or it could be related to a shared environmental cause – pollution from a local factory, for instance. But it certainly does seem that a tendency towards migraine can be inherited: not the headache itself, but some physiological condition which makes migraine possible or more likely. Recent research has isolated a gene which, it is thought, causes a rare form of migraine, so it is perfectly possible that other genes induce other forms of migraine.

You should not, however, feel doomed to a lifetime of migraine attacks merely because your auntie has them; that will not help you to cope with them, let alone to find strategies to avoid them altogether. Your migraines may well be different from those of other family members: less intense, or more responsive to treatment. Nigel's family history is not untypical, although it is extreme. Both his grandmother and father had migraine. Nigel himself still has migraine in his late forties, and all three of his children have also developed migraine. But each case has developed differently, and the condition has shifted and altered from generation to generation.

'I only dimly remember my grandmother's "sick head-aches",' Nigel told me, 'but I can clearly remember how dreadful my father's migraines were. Poor man, he was ill most weeks for days at a time, in appalling pain and retching; yet he held down a complicated job for years – heaven knows how! Nothing seemed to help him at all.'

Nigel's children have been successfully treated and their condition is now much improved, while Nigel, despite having tried most specialist migraine drugs at some stage of his life, now finds that Panadol and sleep work best of all for him, partly because the attacks have, with time, diminished in strength.

AGE AND SEX

It used to be thought that the very young, and the over-sixties, were exempt from migraine attacks. However, although it is unusual, they can and do occur at both stages of life.

As many boys as girls suffer from migraine in childhood, although two in three adult sufferers are women. Migraine attacks do seem to cluster around the stages of life where hormonal changes are at their most active: in the late teens and early twenties, and (especially for women) around the mid- and late forties, and the early fifties. Those seem to be the times when migraine is most likely to strike, or when an earlier migraine pattern may recur after years of freedom from any symptoms.

Most people have their first migraine attack before the age of forty, and most find that the severity and frequency of attacks decline after they reach their mid- to late fifties. And the number of women with migraine is far higher than the number of men, probably because of the high incidence of menstrual, and menstrually related, migraine. But not only is there no justice in migraine, there is also no certainty; predicting the probabilities is almost as difficult as controlling the attacks when they strike.

THE PRICE ON YOUR HEAD

If at least one in ten people suffer from migraine (and, as we've already seen, that figure is probably a conservative one), then in Britain alone, more than six million people are directly affected. Think for a moment about the number of working days that must be lost because of it. A recent figure, estimated from medical certificates giving migraine as the cause, amounted to about one million a year but it has been suggested that a true estimate would be closer to seven million a year. This represents a cost to the nation of about £700 million, every year.

The amount of money spent on drugs to combat migraine is also food for thought. In the United States, more than $500 million is spent each year on headache-relieving drugs, and if only half of that is migraine-related, it still represents a great deal of money, and an awful lot of pills. Migraine is, clearly, a very expensive business.

In a sense, however, those calculations are only the tip of an alarmingly large migraine 'iceberg'. Many people who suffer from migraine conceal that fact from others, perhaps because they fear a lack of sympathy or under-standing, or because they're ashamed of having their lives devastated by 'just a headache'. Others do not realise that their 'sick headaches' or their bouts of nausea, or their visual disturbances, are migraine at all. And many people never consult a doctor about their condition, or do so only rarely. One recent survey showed that only one in two hundred people who said they had headaches ever sought medical advice about them.

'It never struck me that all the bouts of feeling queasy I had for years meant that I might have migraine,' Barbara told me. 'I thought migraine was only a headache, and the headache was never the worst part for me. Now I think of it, I also used to get a sort of flicker in one eye, as well – but I felt so tired, I thought the tiredness was making my eye funny.'

'I couldn't go to the surgery with a *headache*,' explained Margaret. 'They'd just have thought I was a moaning minnie!'

NAMING THE BEAST

Giving something a name is a step on the road to controlling it, just as finding a way to classify headaches is a step towards treating them. The International Headache Society, a neurological organisation, provides the agreed definitions of headaches in general, and migraine in particular.

There are now two main ways of identifying migraine: **migraine without aura** (which used to be called 'common migraine'), and **migraine with aura** (for which the old name was 'classic migraine'). Migraine without aura is by far the more common – it accounts for about 90% of attacks – hence its original name.

Migraine without aura
The three main symptoms of this kind of migraine are the headache itself, the nausea which accompanies it, and a dislike of light. The headache lasts from between four hours to seventy-two hours, and is probably felt on only one side of the head, as a pulsating pain which may well get worse if you move around. The headache may vary from moderate to severe in intensity. If there is also

nausea, it may lead to attacks of vomiting. The other most likely symptom is an increased sensitivity to sound or light, or to both.

Migraine with aura

The main extra symptom of this sort of migraine attack is the aura itself – a visual disturbance of some kind. This can take the form of a blind spot somewhere in the visual field (known as a 'scotoma'), or may be experienced as flashing lights, a general blurring of vision, a zig-zag effect, or even mild hallucinations. These symptoms precede the headache, and typically last for 20 to 30 minutes.

At its most extreme, an aura can cause people to black out and lose consciousness. Other related effects include a numbness which begins in one side of the face or in one arm, and which gradually spreads to other parts of the body. Objects can look larger or smaller, or change shape, or your visual field can break up completely. Many people experiencing these alarming effects for the first time – or who experience them without understanding the cause – believe themselves to be frighteningly ill, or mad, or both.

Other sorts of migraine

Although most of us will always think of a migraine attack as involving a headache at some stage, some people do have migraines with the aura effects, but don't develop a headache! (This used to be called a 'migraine equivalent', but it's now officially classified as a **'migraine aura without headache'**.) Some people who regularly have migraine with auras occasionally have just the aura instead, while others regularly experience only the aura effect.

And there are other, comparatively rare, forms of

14

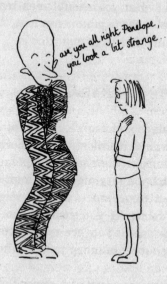

migraine. A **migraine with a prolonged aura** may be diagnosed if the aura lasts for longer than an hour or so. A **basilar migraine** is concentrated on the basilar artery in your brain, and the aura then includes unsteadiness and giddiness, a slurring of speech, hearing problems and double vision. **Abdominal migraine** involves acute pains in your upper abdomen, and is sometimes found in children – as is another uncommon form of migraine called **ophthalmoplegic migraine**, when pain is concentrated around one eye. The pupil of the affected eye becomes dilated, and the eyelid often droops as well. A **retinal migraine** involves a repeated blind spot in one eye or, sometimes, a complete loss of vision in one eye.

All those forms of migraine can be diagnosed and specially treated. But you should seek medical advice if you have any of those symptoms in case they are caused by some problem other than migraine.

OTHER SORTS OF HEADACHE

Not every headache, of course, is migraine-related, and if you get migraine, it unfortunately doesn't mean that you will be free from other sorts of headache in compensation! If you have a late night and a lot of alcohol, you could trigger a migraine – or you might just get a hangover headache. If you swallow an ice-cold drink very quickly, or gobble your ice-cream, you might get an 'ice-cream' headache: a sharp pain at the front of your head.

And headaches *can* warn of a serious abnormality: an impending stroke, for example, or a brain tumour. A progressive increase in the intensity of a headache; or the sudden onset of headaches in someone never before troubled by them; or a sudden, explosive onset of headache; or the alteration of an established headache pattern: all these may be danger signs, and they call for immediate investigation. See your doctor soon if any one of them applies to you.

Cluster headaches
Cluster headaches, once called migrainous neuralgia and thus included within the range of migraine, are now not thought to be migraine at all, although they are still sometimes diagnosed as migraine by doctors, and some experts still prefer to include cluster headaches within a

sort of 'headache continuum', as a very rare version of the migraine condition.

Typically, cluster headaches come in bouts, and occur, say, every day, often at night, for weeks on end. Then there are periods of symptom-free life, with no headaches for weeks, months, or even years. Many patients get cluster headaches at the same time every day, or at the same time every month or even every year. Most sufferers are men, and the pain is often acute, sometimes almost unbearable. Sufferers may bang their heads against the wall in an effort to distract themselves and to relieve the suffering.

Michael, a thirty-seven-year-old teacher, has regularly found himself woken at two in the morning with the agonising pain of a cluster headache. He then walks around the house and garden for hours, trying to shift the focus of his attention away from the pain, usually unsuccessfully. 'I've been on my hands and knees in the garden, weeping with pain,' he said. 'There was so much pressure in my head, I thought half of it would blow off.' Michael has now found relief through drug treatment, but the headaches remain a constant threat in his life.

Tension-type headaches
Tension-type headaches are a very common condition – indeed, something like 80% of people have experienced a tension-type headache at some time in their lives. It can last all day, and for up to a week, and the pain is usually felt on both sides of the head as a tight, pressing sensation. Moving around doesn't make a tension headache worse, and although there may be nausea accompanying it, vomiting doesn't occur. The pain may not be acute, but it often tends to be persistent.

As the name suggests, this sort of headache is thought to be a response to physical or mental tension, stress or anxiety – which may mean that analgesics may not shift the pain. Relaxation exercises of various kinds, however, can be especially effective.

THE NAME OF THE PAIN

You should always go to your doctor first. You may think that your doctor won't be able to help, or you may be so sure that you know the cause of the headaches that medical advice seems unnecessary.

And, of course, you may be right! But your doctor *will* know if the symptoms you have are worth further investigation. Maybe the particular pattern that you experience is similar to some other condition, and in that case your doctor may want to arrange some tests, or a consultation with a specialist. Some headaches are caused by eye infections or by nasal or sinus problems; others may have their origins in dental trouble, or in spinal or muscular strain. These headaches will often respond to treatment, and simple cures may be available.

And if you *do* have migraine, there are more good reasons to seek medical advice. Modern research is providing some real help for the condition, and your GP has access to this information. Perhaps there's a migraine clinic you could attend; or a recent piece of research that throws fresh light on the subject; or a new drug treatment tailor-made for your problem. So don't give up before you've tried your doctor. Asking for help is an important step.

Many people also find that concentrating on listing, and

describing, the symptoms they experience can focus their attention on possible patterns, and that this can help any further investigation. Just the very act of making an appointment to see your GP can set you thinking of possible new connections to be considered and explored. (This is dealt with in detail in Chapter Five.)

IS IT OR IS IT NOT MIGRAINE?

The following checklist is only a guide, and if you think your symptoms match up, it makes excellent sense to have that diagnosis confirmed by your doctor.

★ Do you have any idea that the headache is coming, before it starts to hurt?
★ Is the pain centred on only one side of your head?
★ Is the pain a throbbing one at any stage?
★ Does the pain get worse if you move your head?
★ Does treatment with hot or cold packs relieve the pain?
★ Do you feel queasy, or 'liverish', with the headache?
★ Do you feel so nauseous you want to vomit – and perhaps do so?
★ Do you want to lie down, be left alone, and avoid noise and light?
★ Do you notice differences in your sense of smell?
★ Is the pain so bad you feel you want to cry?
★ Do you see flashes or zig-zags of light at the sides of your eyes, or get a blind spot in your vision?
★ Does your arm or face, or the side of your body, tingle or go numb?
★ Do you look unusually pale, or drawn?

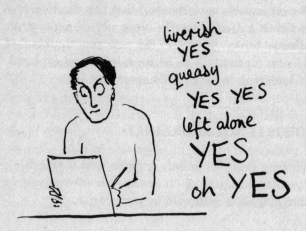

★ Does the experience last for between two hours and three days?

Not everyone with migraine has more than two of those symptoms; some very unfortunate people have all of them. The essential symptoms for a sure medical diagnosis are the (usually one-sided) headache, and some form of accompanying nausea or dislike of light, but the headache can shift, and the nausea can vary in intensity. And some people have different sorts of migraine at different times of their lives.

Seeing the pattern
Migraine symptoms do tend to form a pattern. It may be very difficult to identify the pattern, and it may vary from one attack to another. But it will be there, and if you persist, with time, help and care you will first be able to identify it, and then learn to recognise the stages.

Sometimes, the symptoms will be fairly obvious; they may be common ones, or ones which you share with other members of your family. But others may be less obvious, or unexpected.

'I never realised that my sudden frequent need to pee had anything to do with my migraine,' said one sufferer I interviewed. 'When I discovered that other people had identified that as part of the "hangover" phase of an attack, I felt really pleased – as though I had one more piece of evidence to add to the puzzle-solving.'

THE MIGRAINE'S PROGRESS

There are five stages of a migraine attack. Not everyone will experience them all, but it is well worth considering each of the stages to see if you recognise any of the symptoms, or if you might be able to learn to do so. Sometimes it is easier for others to spot the signs than for the sufferers themselves – so if you can, enlist help! This is especially valuable for the first warning stage; if you or your friends and family can learn to identify your warning signs, and if you then act fast with effective remedies, you will be able to avoid the worst of the attack – or even avoid it altogether.

1. Stage one: the warning signs (called the 'prodrome')
The early signs of an impending migraine attack typically come the day before – or the evening before – the headache begins. Sometimes the signs take the form of a change of mood: some people become especially irritable, while others feel elated and unusually cheerful. You

might feel suddenly filled with energy, or very light-hearted and jokey. Another common symptom is a sudden craving for a particular food, often for something sweet, like chocolate. Or you may feel unusually tired, and find yourself yawning and sighing a lot; or feel muddle-headed and clumsy, unable to express yourself clearly or compose your thoughts. You may feel bloated or constipated or have diarrhoea, or you may find you urinate more or less than usual.

'I feel very tired just before an attack,' Fiona told me, 'as though my brain and my body are wading through treacle, and they're not even in step! It's a lot like the feeling I get when I'm fighting off a cold or flu, and it took me ages to learn the difference.'

'Typically,' said Jean, 'I have a great surge of energy the night before. It's as if I've been under the weather, and suddenly I feel really terrific – as though I could fight tigers! But I have learned to connect that – if it comes out of the blue – to waking up with a migraine the next morning, and so I can prepare myself. Sometimes, if I take pain-killers when I go to bed the night before, I can avoid the worst of the migraine starting up at all.'

'I sometimes get a sort of twinkle in my eye,' explained Hannah. 'I used to ignore it, or just screw up my eyes to get rid of it: I thought it was a sort of blip in my focus. Now I know what it means!'

2. Stage two: the aura
This stage usually develops quite slowly, and seldom lasts for more than an hour. The headache, if it comes, generally arrives after it. The aura often takes the form of visual disturbances, but many people also experience numbness in their face or other parts of their body, or a

general tingling or clumsiness. Some people see flashing lights, or a 'zig-zag' effect at the side of their visual field. Others experience a blind spot in their vision – the 'bagel' effect – which may spread and vary in size and shape, before it fades away. Sometimes the whole visual field blacks out, or just parts of it, so that the sufferer can only see straight ahead.

'The first one I ever had gave me very blurred vision,' said Fiona. 'I was wearing glasses, and I realised that there was a whole bit of the world I couldn't see through them. I thought it was the glasses, but when I took them off, I *still* couldn't see properly.'

The aura effect tends to advance slowly. Scott, typically, will realise only gradually that something is odd about what he is seeing. 'It's as though something's missing,' he explained. 'I'll be looking at someone's face, say, and then it seems as though the lighting has dimmed and I can't see the person clearly any more.'

Philip, a hairdresser, has also had trouble seeing people's faces clearly during a migraine attack, but sometimes the effects move quickly. 'I glanced at a client in the mirror just last week,' he told me, 'and it was as if the whole bottom half of her face had been wiped out! I usually have more warning of an aura than that, and I almost asked her if there was something wrong with her mouth before I realised it was me, not her. I simply had to stop work and walk away – luckily, I'd finished cutting by then!'

Unsurprisingly, this stage can be a terrifying one to experience. Even migraineurs who have been having attacks for years can still dread the appearance of the aura – not only because they fear what will follow, but also because the aura itself is so unsettling.

3. Stage three: the headache and nausea

The essence of the migraine attack is focused on this main stage – the headache itself, and the related symptoms of nausea, vomiting, and avoidance of light and noise. Typically, a migraine headache begins when you wake up, perhaps as a dull and non-specific ache which gradually becomes more acute over time. Sometimes people dream of having a migraine, and wake to find it's true. Oliver Sacks recounts dreaming of people with bits of their faces missing – and waking with a migraine in full swing.

Sometimes the pain remains as a constant ache, which increases to a throbbing pain if you have to move around. Any movement often increases the pain, which makes the nausea and vomiting especially distressing. The pain might radiate down your neck to your shoulder, and perhaps even to your arm and leg as well, on the same side of your body.

Sometimes the very smell or even the thought of food can increase the nausea and induce vomiting; sometimes vomiting continues until the patient is just retching repeatedly, without bringing anything up. In some cases, the vomiting stage is quickly followed by the migraineur beginning to feel better; the vomiting can bring stage three to an end. For others, unfortunately, that is not the case, and there is more to come.

Another common symptom of stage three is the dislike of light and noise, and an acute desire to hide away from other people. Someone with a migraine seldom wants sympathy and attention from other people, even if they would usually like them in normal circumstances.

Certain smells sometimes become intolerable, and for some people a dislike of particular smells can even be an early warning sign. Even some smells which are generally considered pleasant, such as particular perfumes, can be implicated.

'I remember once taking refuge in the spare room during a migraine attack,' said Kate, one migraine sufferer. 'I had a bowl of pot-pourri in there to keep the room fresh, and it was a mixture I loved. But that day, the smell seemed ten times as strong as I'd noticed before, and it became really offensive to me. It seemed to leave a sort of after-taste – or after-smell – in my nose, and made the headache and the nausea much worse. And now, I've had to change the mixture; I hate the reminder, and I'm scared it will bring a migraine on.'

A generally increased sensitivity can mean that even a

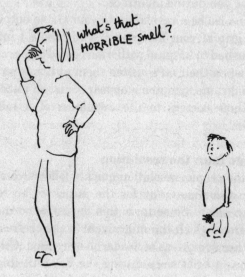

softly ticking clock, a mere crack of light, or even low-voiced speech can seem a dreadful imposition. Speech, and coherent thought, are often impaired – some people find that they cannot easily form sentences, or recall simple details of their life or work. Others report an increased nasal 'stuffiness'. I always have an alternately blocked or running left nostril throughout this part of a migraine attack, and when it clears, I know the attack is almost over. It is as though the migraineur's whole nervous system becomes especially vulnerable.

Many people *look* very ill indeed when they are in this stage of a migraine. Sunken (and later, even bruised) eyes and a complete lack of colour are common. All that, combined with dizziness or numbness in the arms and legs, can be very alarming for your family and friends if they see you during an attack.

It can also be a revelation to your GP to encounter you in the grip of your symptoms. Two people I interviewed were rushed to hospital with a suspected cerebral haemorrhage when their GPs visited them at home, so acute did their migraine symptoms appear – and so unaccustomed were their doctors to the awfulness of a migraine in progress!

4. Stage four: the resolution

For some people, resolution quickly follows vomiting, but the most common way for the attack to be resolved is through sleep. Sometimes this is just a normal night's sleep, from which the migraineur wakes refreshed, with no further symptoms of headache or nausea. Other people find that a brief sleep during the day will do the trick. Some can achieve a resolution by sleeping or just dozing for as little as fifteen minutes, but most people find that at least a couple of hours is necessary.

'If I manage to take pain-killers in time – and for me, just a regular over-the-counter analgesic like ibuprofen will do the trick if I catch it early – then I can sleep it off in three or four hours,' said one sufferer. A proper sleep, rather than just a snooze, seems to be the best, but some find that a short rest will damp down the symptoms sufficiently for them to finish with the day's demands. A good night's sleep then completes the process. However, this is not always true. The headache can wax and wane, gradually losing strength, and only truly disappear with the passage of time, perhaps after several days.

5. Stage five: the 'hangover' (called the 'post-drome')
Feeling some sort of hangover effect after a migraine attack is very common. For many people this takes the form of feeling weak and washed out, generally tired and debilitated. This can last for just a few hours – perhaps for the rest of the day on which the headache ends – or it can last for three or four days afterwards. Migraineurs who describe this hangover effect talk of being less efficient in their jobs, or being tired despite lots of early nights and resting. 'I get really depressed about that part,' one told me. 'I've been through the hell of throwing up and having that crashing pain, but then I *still* feel awful, like a piece of used elastic.'

Some people find that treating their migraine with drugs intensifies a 'down' effect for them in the hangover period. If they leave the migraine to run its course without taking drugs, they know they will suffer the full pain and discomfort of the worst of the attack, but they will also have the benefit of an easier and quicker resolution.

'It's like being caught between the devil and the deep

blue sea!' said one man who uses Sanomigran to prevent recurrent migraine attacks. 'The pills do work, but I feel woozy and odd too much of the time, and I've put on weight from the pills, as well.'

For some people, the hangover after-effect takes a very different shape. Once the headache and nausea are over, these migraineurs wake to an intensely vibrant world, with a heightened sense of awareness and energy – just as other sufferers feel in the warning stage of an attack.

'I could take on the world when the headache's gone,' said one person. 'I can charge through everything that's piled up on my desk while I was sick, in half the time it would usually take me. I feel really special: like myself, but more so.'

One man, whose migraines have now gone, described that sensation as 'the most intensely creative times of my life. I dreaded each migraine attack and loathed the pain and the vomiting, but at least I knew that those golden days were coming afterwards – when I could do anything I wanted.'

The simple relief that the dreadful symptoms are over can also bring a great feeling of elation and well-being to the thankful sufferer.

CHAPTER 2

What's Happening in My Head?

Any theory about the causes of migraine has to account for a wide range of symptoms, which vary greatly amongst migraineurs. The stages of a migraine, and the attacks themselves, have been carefully described, and lists of potential triggers have been developed. But the discussions about what *causes* the attacks are still going on.

Agreement about what happens – at least in broad terms – is now more or less certain amongst the scientific experts. But determining which is cause and which are effects is quite another matter! Some experts argue in favour of one factor being the cause; others argue in favour of another. Still others support the idea that a collection of factors working together is the real cause.

PUZZLING IT OUT

One of the most curious things about migraine is the involvement of pain, when no serious disease is involved. Pain is usually a sign that something is wrong; serious pain is usually a sign of something seriously wrong. If migraine isn't life-threatening, why does it hurt so much?

And there are many other puzzles about migraine to keep the experts busy. Why do some people suffer from migraine, while others do not? After all, only a very few people can truthfully report (no doubt with a certain tone of superiority) that they have *never* had any kind of headache. Some things – acute tension and anxiety, for example, or very bright light, or drinking and smoking – *often* produce headaches in many, maybe even most, people. But for just a few, those events produce a full-blown migraine. Why doesn't everyone get migraine? (Or better still, why doesn't everyone *not* get it?) Why is the headache one-sided? What on earth is going on inside your head – and the rest of your body – during a migraine attack?

In order to understand any of this, we are going to have to look at some of the processes that go on in human bodies. You don't have to have a medical background to take in the main ideas that are involved, and once you get the hang of them, the explanations are fascinating. It's like opening a door into a secret world – that's all happening inside *you*!

THE USES OF PAIN

Pain is usually a protective device. Our bodies use it to avoid damage. If you touch a hot stove, the pain makes you whip your hand away, and so you avoid getting a serious burn. If you sprain your ankle, the pain makes you stop putting your full weight on the ankle until it has a chance to recover.

Pain is caused by messages which are sent along the nerve fibres in your body. Most of the nerves in your body produce a sensation of pain by increasing the frequency of the messages they send. If you touch a stove that's just pleasantly warm, the nerves in your hand will send messages quite slowly through your hand and arm to your spinal cord. If the heat increases, the frequency of the messages increases as well. If the heat is intense enough to cause a burn, the nerves fire off messages rapidly and continuously, and that burst of activity registers as pain in your central nervous system.

So the device of pain is very useful to your body, but the nerves which set it off can also be stimulated in other ways, and produce misery instead of protection. If your brain's pain-control system isn't working properly, you can feel what's called 'spontaneous pain' – pain without a physical cause. This may be one of the factors involved in headaches.

Pain in your head can be caused by the nerves which report sensations in your scalp, or in the muscles and bones in your neck and skull. Some of the pain of migraine is also thought to be produced by the nerves which surround the walls of the arteries bringing blood to your face and scalp and brain, because the symptoms of migraine involve temporary alterations to the blood vessels in your head. So let's put the nerve question to one side for a moment, and look at the way your blood vessels work.

BLOOD LINES

An adult human body contains about five litres of blood. This travels around through a complicated system of tubes: arteries, capillaries, and veins. The main tubes are the arteries, and these are surrounded with nerve fibres and muscles which respond to changes in pressure as the blood is pumped by your heart through your body.

The jacket of muscles around an artery contracts and relaxes all the time to regulate the blood flow (the blood pressure), and to control the way in which blood is distributed to various parts of your body. In physical exercise, for instance, more blood flows through the arteries to the capillaries which supply your lungs; after a meal, more blood is pumped to your digestive organs.

Blood on the brain

Your brain, like the other organs in your body, needs a regular supply of blood. It needs to receive oxygen and sugar to do its tasks efficiently, and once its tasks are completed, it needs to dispose of waste materials like carbon dioxide.

The human brain is well supplied with blood by four main arteries. Each of these carries blood not only to the brain, but also to the outside of the skull. And in the first stages of a migraine attack, the branches of the blood vessels inside your skull contract. Then, as the headache develops, the branches outside your skull dilate, usually only on one side of your head. Sometimes you can see them standing out around the area of pain. The arteries become so sensitive that any variation in blood pressure sends off waves of pain messages from the artery walls.

In a **migraine with aura** attack, there is a reduction in the amount of blood which flows to the brain. The decrease usually starts at the back of the brain, and moves forward quite slowly.

There is a minimum amount of blood which your brain needs to function properly, and if the blood supply drops below that level, certain symptoms will – and do – occur. These symptoms typically begin in the occipital lobes, which are at the base of your skull, just as it curves out and away from your neck. The occipital lobes are in charge of vision: that's why visual disturbances often herald the aura of a migraine. If the blood supply further forward in your brain also drops, then numbness and weakness in your face, arms and legs will occur – and all of these are familiar aura symptoms for many migraine patients.

The timing of the reduction in blood supply and the onset of the aura are not always consistent. Sometimes the blood flow drops before the aura begins, and continues at a low level after the aura has ended. But in most cases which have been studied, the timing of the reduced blood supply is matched to the symptoms of the aura, and so the theoretical link has been made.

However, the results are not as clear for **migraine without aura**. Sometimes the migraine headache follows an increased blood supply to the brain, but sometimes the headache cannot be linked to any increase in blood flow. So there may be an important difference between these two main sorts of migraine.

Now, since the pain involved in these changes is carried by nerves, we can return to the story of the nerves, and how they work. Don't go away – the climax of the story will soon be revealed!

LOTS OF NERVE

The nerve that carries sensations from your face and the front two-thirds of your scalp is called the trigeminal nerve – the 'tri' part of the name means it has three divisions. This is the nerve involved in most of the pain of migraine, for it is not only in charge of messages about your forehead, cheek and chin, but it also controls the messages which come from the nerves which jacket the blood vessels in your brain.

When an artery becomes distended, its jacketing network of nerve fibres stretch as well, and give off messages that they are doing so. These messages register as pain. If the messages increase with each pulse of your heart, they register as a throbbing pain. If the arteries inside your skull become dilated, the pain gets worse when you move, because the arteries have come into contact with the highly sensitive tissue which surrounds your brain. All of these effects are involved in a migraine headache. And there's more . . .

The pathways and the gates

The message along a nerve is carried in two different ways: by electricity, and by chemicals. At first, the message is sent by an electrical impulse moving along the nerve fibres from section to section.

But the message needs to get from one section of the nerve to the next in order to reach the central nervous system – and there are gaps which separate one section from another, rather like gates along a path. The pain message must jump over the gates.

To help the message jump the gates, the first section of the nerve releases chemicals which attract the attention of the next section of the nerve pathway, and tells it to send the wave of electricity, with its pain message, on down the line.

And it is here, at the gateways, that migraine seems to have its origins. We have reached the heart of the mystery, and the reasons behind the misery. It all seems to be contained in the balance of ingredients here, in a sort of chemical soup, and the way that the balance of chemicals in the soup is achieved.

P is for pain

Chemicals released by nerve fibres are neuro-transmitters: they transmit nerve messages. One sort of neuro-transmitter involved in pain is a peptide called 'Substance P'. When the peptide is released, the tiny nerve cells which control the gateway respond by releasing other chemicals, and the sorts they release, and the amounts they release, determine whether or not the pain message is transmitted. These chemicals are like pain *control* guards at the gateway.

The guard transmitters ensure either that messages are passed on, or that they are blocked. The guards can mask the message so the pain is reduced or ignored. They can also reduce the efficiency of the next section of the pathway, so that it doesn't send the message on very quickly. What the guards *actually* do depends on what instructions they receive. In migraineurs, these instructions seem to depend on the levels of one particular chemical, called **serotonin**.

There are a number of other chemicals which your body uses in the nerve gateways. Some are enzymes which speed up chemical reactions, and destroy any transmitter substances that are not used up or reabsorbed. But the neuro-transmitters which are thought to be crucial to migraine are called amines – chemicals with an amine as part of their structure.

Your body produces lots of amines (adrenalin, noradrenalin and dopamine, for example, are all amines), but the one which has dominated the migraine research spotlight for the last few years – and which will probably continue to do so for some time to come – is serotonin. It is a monoamine ('mono' because, like noradrenalin, it contains only one amine), and it is sometimes referred to by its chemical name: 5-hydroxytryptamine, or 5HT for short.

Serotonin: a starring role

Serotonin is a neuro-transmitter, and it influences the pain messages your nerves send. But that is not its only job in your body. In fact, serotonin acts in many different places in your body, and affects the receiving and sending of a host of different sorts of messages. There are receptors for serotonin at many sites – four different sorts of serotonin receptors have so far been identified.

If all this sounds confusing, don't worry – you are not alone! Scientists, too, are confused about exactly what serotonin does, and how it does it. But although not all of its functions are yet identified or understood, one thing seems clear: serotonin makes the blood vessels in your brain and scalp swell up and cause pain.

Migraine experts now know that serotonin is released into your bloodstream before a migraine headache begins, and makes the blood vessels swell. Then, when the pain messages arrive at the gateways, the pain control system – the guards at the gateways – seems to break down.

Have the chemical guards gone off-duty, or have they

been defeated by some other chemical? Have they been transferred to another post, or to other duties? Whatever the reason, the serotonin levels have dropped, affecting your body's normal control of blood vessels.

It may be that migraineurs produce unusual levels (either too much or too little) of serotonin. It may be that we process such amines less effectively than other people, or perhaps our nervous systems are somehow more sensitive to serotonin and other monoamines. We may have a factor in our blood which makes serotonin storage sites release their deposits. Maybe our enzyme levels are different, or more easily disturbed. All these questions still need answers.

But the importance of all this is that it has helped scientists to develop new drugs which combat the migrainous effects of serotonin. They have designed drugs to mimic specific actions of serotonin – or to block those actions. Some of these drugs work better than others; some work well for some people and not so well for other people. Perhaps that means that the *real* effects of serotonin on migraine are still to be identified . . .

Why, why, why . . .
But where does all this serotonin activity begin – and why does it start up at all? There are three main theories.

1. It might begin in the blood vessels themselves.

2. It might begin with the release of serotonin into your bloodstream, affecting your blood vessels and the way your brain controls pain.

3. Or it could start in the brain, which could itself determine the release of serotonin to your nerve pathways and your blood vessels.

The idea that migraine is a disorder of the blood vessels

is the oldest theory still in current use today. Most scientists agree that migraine can be described as a 'vascular headache': a headache linked to changes in the blood vessels. The vessels become constricted and narrow, and then dilate, expanding to more than their usual size. No one doubts that changes in the blood vessels occur during migraine attacks. But whether these changes cause migraine, or are themselves the result of other causes, is disputed. Blood vessels can – and do – shut down for their own reasons; but is that true in migraine?

BUT THEN AGAIN . . .

Research into migraine is constantly throwing up new theories about possible causes.

The role of platelets
Platelets are tiny cells which circulate in the bloodstream, and are usually responsible for repairing any faults in the lining of blood vessels. Their ability to stick together and form clumps is the first stage in the clotting process which mends gaps in cut or damaged blood vessels.

One of the chemicals which platelets release into your bloodstream is serotonin, and so the role of platelets has come under close scrutiny in recent studies. One school of thought believes that the platelets themselves are directly responsible for causing migraine attacks.

Histamine
It is not only neuro-transmitters like serotonin which have been studied for their possible role in migraine. Histamine, a chemical which human bodies produce in

response to physical shock or injury, and during an allergic reaction, also affects the contraction and dilation of blood vessels. Although the scientific evidence so far remains unclear, many migraineurs find relief from their symptoms by using anti-histamine drugs in combination with other drugs. And the belief that migraine is primarily an allergic response – especially to foods – is a strong one amongst some people.

Blood-sugar levels

Your body needs glucose like a car needs petrol, but it has to keep the levels of glucose in your bloodstream at a fairly steady level. The levels should not rise too high, nor fall too low: both are potentially dangerous conditions.

If you eat a potato, your body will convert the carbohydrate into glucose, and it will do so quite slowly, over several hours. If you eat a toffee, the conversion of sugar into glucose happens much faster – a matter of minutes.

After it reaches your bloodstream, the glucose is absorbed in different ways. Some of it remains in the blood, to provide an immediate source of energy. Some of it is stored in muscles and in the liver, as a substance called glycogen, which can rapidly be converted back into glucose. Excess glucose is converted into fat, which is stored in the body. It, too, can be transformed back into energy, but not as quickly, or as readily, as can the glycogen, which your body will automatically use up first.

Nervous tissue has no store of glycogen, so the cells in your nervous tissue have to rely on the glucose which circulates in the blood. If the blood supply of glucose drops too low – for example, if you have low blood sugar – you may trigger a migraine. (Low blood sugar – the medical name is hypoglycaemia – has other unpleasant side-effects too: tiredness, irritability, confusion, and so on. Prolonged fasting can cause it, or heavy exercise; and it can also occur in diabetics if they take an overdose of insulin.)

There seems to be a frequent connection between low blood-sugar levels and migraine. Migraine attacks often cease, or become less frequent, during periods of rapid weight gain and in pregnancy: times of relatively high blood-sugar levels. Migraine attacks often begin in the morning, a time when blood-sugar levels tend to be low.

Some migraine sufferers are liable to develop a migraine if they skip a meal, or if a meal is delayed. The same thing can happen if a migraineur 'sleeps in' late, and so delays a meal – although it's hard to identify the exact trigger in such cases. Fatty foods, too, are often cited as triggers for migraine, and eating fatty foods can provoke big swings in blood-sugar levels, as can eating sugary things.

I'm not just a symptom

In the middle of all this science, however, it's important to remember there's a person: a human being, whose existence is more than the chemistry of nervous energy or the metabolism of sugar. Migraine is a disorder which arises from the relationship between your central nervous system and your body's health and well-being – but your feelings and desires, your imagination and your most cherished beliefs, your creativity, and your responses to the world in which you live, all also play an essential part.

CHAPTER 3

Where Does it Spring From?

Trying to identify exactly what brings on a migraine attack can be a bewildering task. Migraine clearly involves a wide range of factors, and sorting these out takes patience as well as time.

In the last chapter, I summarised the current theories about the physiological and neurological *causes* of migraine, and the evidence which has been gathered to support those ideas. But in this chapter, the focus is on practical ideas closer to home. Why do some people get migraine and others not? What triggers the attacks?

KNOWLEDGE IS POWER

If you want to learn to manage your migraines – to attack the problem in an active and successful way – then you will need to understand something of the reasons behind migraine. And although you can (and should) involve the medical profession in this, it also makes excellent sense to put yourself in command by appointing yourself the general in charge of the battle! After all, no one else will ever care as much as you do about the things which are happening to *you*.

A THREE-PART PROGRAMME

There are three basic ways to sort out what brings on a migraine attack.

1. Look at the theories

The first way is to assess the **theories** about who gets migraine, and to see if the evidence helps you to identify a pattern in your own attacks.

If you understand a little of why you get migraine, you may also feel more comfortable and less confused about it. You may stop blaming yourself – and stop others from trying to do so – if you can point to the real reasons for your migraines.

The first part of this chapter outlines some of the ideas about *why* migraine strikes.

2. Beware the warning signs

The second way is to think carefully about **warning signs**: the clues which show that a migraine attack has been precipitated, and that the first stage, the 'prodrome', has already begun. If you are lucky enough to recognise your own warning signs, you may be able to prevent the attack from happening, or to avoid its worst effects. (Go back and have another look at pages 21 to 22, if you have forgotten the sort of clues you should be searching for.)

3. Pinpoint your trigger factors

And the third way is to look closely at the **trigger factors**: the likely reasons for the attack to begin. If you know what your trigger factors are, you stand an excellent chance of avoiding attacks. The second half of this chapter concentrates on listing possible trigger factors, and on helping you to identify your own.

WHY ME?

The evidence from people who have reported their migraine experiences to doctors, and those who have been involved in migraine studies over the years, shows a 'likelihood' profile of typical migraineurs.

What do migraineurs have in common?

If everyone who experienced migraine attacks shared just one or two characteristics – or even if most of them did – then discovering *why* they suffered in this way would be much more straightforward. A cause would be much more obvious. A cure would be much more likely to be identified.

But the 'likelihood' picture is much more complicated. Migraine is a very complex human disorder, and simple patterns are not easily found within it. People who have migraine attacks clearly share *that* experience, but do they all share something else, too? And if it's not an obvious thing they share – like blue eyes, or a passion for baroque organ music – then is there some other *hidden* factor which underlies their attacks?

A secret pathway through your defences?

The most popular explanation amongst modern experts is that migraineurs share a physiological **predisposition**. That means that the nervous systems of people who get migraine respond to particular events in a different way from other people. And the way in which migraineurs respond, it is thought, leads to the pattern of the migraine attack.

The argument goes like this. Suppose that you have inherited an *ability* for migraine from your father. And suppose that inheritance makes your nervous system especially sensitive to a combination of emotional stress, a flickering TV screen, and a particular additive in take-away food. In that case, the first time you sit down to a TV dinner after a shouting-match with your boss, you may well also develop your first migraine!

Learning to have a migraine

An analogy used by one expert compares the way your body 'learns' to have a migraine attack, to the way in which you learn how to ride a bicycle. The pattern of coordinated movements for bicycle riding, once learned, is not forgotten; people who have not biked for years can do so again in a few moments, without a refresher course. They don't have to think about it, either; they can just do it. The sight of the bicycle somehow keys their muscles, their nerves, and their brain to respond in a particular pattern. The pathway of response has been laid down.

So, migraine might work in the same way. Migraineurs have nervous systems in which pathways of response have been laid down. Their nervous systems have become highly susceptible to a particular circumstance, or to particular combinations of circumstances. Given those circumstances, certain responses are triggered, and the attack begins.

Of course, this model does not explain what factors decide who gets a migraine attack in the first place, and who does not. But it does provide a useful background.

Times of high risk

Studies conducted at one British hospital have revealed definite 'peak periods' in a lifetime for experiencing migraine. For women, it was found, migraine attacks typically happened in bouts between the ages of nine and eleven, between seventeen and eighteen, and in the early forties. Men, however, typically experienced migraine attacks between thirteen and fifteen, in their mid-twenties, and in their late forties to early fifties. It is rare to suffer migraine attacks regularly throughout your life. Most people's experiences of migraine tend to clump together, with periods of few or no attacks lasting for months or even years.

Me and my hormones

Since those peak periods are all times of disturbance in hormone levels, it is suggested that hormone alterations may act as 'sensitisers' for migraine. If you carry the capacity for migraine around in your body, then one way for a pathway to be established is through an alteration in hormone levels. And, once your nervous system has been sensitised in that way, other factors can use the established pathway to produce the same effect. It is as though a hidden tendency has been unmasked.

Menstruation and migraines

Since migraine is more likely to occur in women than in men, it is not surprising that many female migraineurs identify a relationship between their menstrual cycle and their migraine attacks. Many women experience their first migraine around the time when they have their first period. For some women, migraine attacks seem to diminish once the menstrual cycle is established, but it may also return – especially if they use contraceptive pills.

If this pattern sounds familiar to you, you may already know that migraine usually disappears during pregnancy – more than 80% of pregnant migraineurs lose their migraines after the first few months. Some women also stop having migraines when they begin the menopause, but for others this is a time of increased migraine activity. (There's more about this hormone connection on pages 72 to 74.)

Good times, bad times
Many migraineurs who have tried to learn to identify the pattern of their migraine attacks know that there are times when they can eat 'danger list' foods, drink red wine, and stay up late with complete impunity. No migraine attacks arrive, no matter how many triggers they have pulled! Many say that this happens immediately after a migraine attack. It is as though their systems have been somehow 'emptied' of migraine.

Some people learn to develop an awareness of such patterns, and to use the knowledge to plan for the immediate 'safe' future. But a long migraine-free period can be worrying, since it can seem as though the attack is building up strength in some mysterious way.

'Every three months or so, I seem to get a real corker,' Jean explained. 'And they only come if I've had a longer break than usual between ordinary migraines.'

For some women, the migraine threshold is lowered by hormone changes: in the week before a period, for example. Or you may find that if you're tired, or feeling depressed, or especially stressed, you are more likely to get a migraine. It's at such times that trigger factors must be monitored meticulously, and that you must put into practice all you've learned.

Unfair, unfair . . .

Of course, most people in the world do *not* have a migraine attack when their bodies are filled with hormone disturbances, nor when they are leading an especially stressful life. No lists of suspect foods need to litter their kitchens or stretch their cooking skills to the limit; no complicated label-reading needs to delay their shopping expeditions; no diary entries have to track the passage of events like a military historian . . .

Feeling different and isolated – and somehow 'picked on' by fate – can be a serious problem for migraine sufferers, especially if they know no others in a similar position. That's why support groups, self-help organisations, and associations like the British Migraine Association are such a life-line for many people. 'I'd never met anyone else like me before,' one member of the Leicester Migraine Self-Help Group told me. 'I used to spend my time feeling confused and depressed, and setting up problems all the time. Now I have all the support and understanding in the world, and I can spend my time looking for solutions, instead of problems!'

TRIGGER-HAPPY

The range of potential triggers for a migraine attack is large, but if you group them into 'families' of related probability, you can begin to make sense of the task.

The Leicester Migraine Self-Help Group divides potential triggers into groups, and the chart which follows is based on one which they issue to their members. It is a very useful place to begin your search.

It *is* only a first step – tracking down your own triggers may well involve you in more complicated note-keeping – but even just reading through the chart will focus your attention on the areas to consider. Sometimes, only a small adjustment will do it – the trick is to identify that one small thing . . .

Migraine Trigger Chart

	Migraines				
Emotional stress factors	1	2	3	4	5
anger					
anxiety					
boredom					
change of job					
excitement					
holiday					
shock					
stress					
post-stress					
(add your own personal ideas)					
Physical and environmental factors					
bending or stooping					
change of climate or altitude					
hospitalisation					
late rising					
muscle tension					
over-exertion or sudden exercise					
shift work					
travel					
very hot bath					
(add your own personal ideas)					

		Migraines			
Physiological factors	1	2	3	4	5
bright or glaring light					
contraceptive pills					
loud noises					
menopause					
menstruation					
sleeping pills					
smells					
smoking					
visual disturbances eg. flickering lights, pattern disturbances					
(add your own personal ideas)					
Food factors					
alcohol					
cheese					
chocolate					
citrus fruit					
coffee and tea					
dairy products					
fasting or dieting					
food additives (eg. monosodium glutamate)					
fried foods					
irregular meals					
(add your own personal ideas)					

Using the trigger chart

The chart is an excellent and simple place to start. When you next have a migraine (or if you have just had one in the past few days), tick off all the factors that could be applied to it. Think about the day which preceded the attack as well.

Then do the same thing with your next migraine attack – and the one after that. By now, you will have a better idea of what is *not* an issue for you, and you can probably begin to discount certain things, and to look more closely at others. You will be able to begin to build up a possible pattern of trigger factors to consider.

And the process of considering all these possibilities will also start to make you more aware – of yourself, and your life-style. Next time, you will be able to add specific potential triggers to this list of general ones, and check your ideas of what may be true against what seems to be true.

Thinking it through

I firmly believe that *no* time is better spent by a migraineur than in trying to identify potential trigger factors. The difficulty comes when you feel confused, or reach a dead-end, and need help to find a new direction, or to sort it all out.

It is an exceptional GP who is able to spend time talking these things through with you, or who will have enough detailed knowledge to be helpful (most medical students get only one half-hour lecture on migraine during their training). The doctors attached to migraine clinics *are* experts in the field, but not all clinics allow time for such discussion, or are able to give you such an appointment when you need it.

51

A support group, if one is available to you, is an invaluable resource of patience and knowledge. So is the constant stream of members' suggestions with which the British Migraine Association's newsletters are filled. (This is also a source of information about local support groups – and somewhere to advertise if you want to set one up.)

Once again, you are fortunate if you have a sympathetic partner or family member who will help in your search. Sometimes the obvious is *not* obvious to the person themselves: it was my partner who pointed out to me the coincidence of my migraines and my period, the last time I suffered badly with migraine attacks. The link had been staring me in the face but I just didn't see it!

Where do you start?
So many potential triggers are related to food and food consumption, or to hormones, that those are both excellent places to begin. In fact, **food consumption** – especially the timing of meals – is probably the strongest trigger of all.

FOOD FOR THOUGHT

Identifying particular foods which trigger migraine has been an established method of treatment for some years. Most people now know that certain foods – **cheese** and **red wine** are probably the most infamous – are said to be especially likely to bring on an attack. If you avoid the foods on the standard migraine list, the argument goes, you can also avoid migraine attacks.

Well, that sounds straightforward, doesn't it? And I wish it *were* that easy for everyone. But it isn't. Migraine, alas, is not a simple condition – and so trying to avoid certain foods may not work for you. Perhaps you aren't being ruthless about excluding *every* source of the food. Perhaps there's more than one food trigger involved, and you've only managed to identify one of them. Perhaps you're mistaken about the food, and you've identified the wrong one. Or, perhaps, you just don't have any food triggers at all . . . Help!

But that does *not* mean you shouldn't try! You should; most people who have managed to alleviate or stop their migraines completely have done so through searching for food-related triggers. But it does mean you should work out a sensible way of approaching the business.

Food triggers: dos and don'ts

1. Don't give up all the suggested triggers at once. The list is a long one, and you'll end up miserable, with far too restricted a diet for health or sense, and very likely creating more migraine problems for yourself through stress or by yo-yoing your blood-sugar levels.

If you don't know where to start but you're desperate to have a go, begin with one of the most common ones. Look back at the food factors section of the trigger chart, and choose one that featured at or around the time of your last migraine.

2. Do pick one food, or one food group, and make sure you are cutting it out *completely*. Some things – like **chocolate** and **caffeine** – are hidden ingredients in other products. **Monosodium glutamate** is not only used by most Chinese restaurants (the menu will often tell you if they *don't* use it, but not if they do), it also appears under different names in a lot of processed food: as 621; as MSG; as Aji-no-moto. You don't just need to take your glasses to

the supermarket to read the labels – you need a code-breaker as well!

3. Do remember that giving up certain foods can produce unpleasant side-effects for a few days. You will probably get withdrawal effects if you drink more than just one cup of tea or coffee a day, and then give it up: the caffeine in these is a drug to which your body becomes accustomed. You may even get a bad headache – or a migraine – in those few days.

The final effects of giving up may very well be worth enduring the transition miseries for, but if you are prepared for the possible unpleasantness, you are much more likely to succeed.

4. Don't let the restriction in your diet lead to skipping meals. Low blood-sugar levels, or delayed meals, can in themselves be migraine triggers.

5. Do remember that you can experiment with reintroducing a food if it doesn't seem to be the culprit after all – or if you suspect that certain forms of the food may be safe for you. Some people find, for example, that cooked cheese is a certain trigger but that other cheeses are safe.

6. Don't feel you have to *prove* you've found the trigger by trying to behave like a laboratory scientist! If you're convinced that nuts have been the culprit and you're happy to do without them, that's great – congratulations! It's only if your nut-exclusion hasn't really worked that you might want to modify things. Could it have been the salt, or a colouring or preservative in your chosen brand? And might that be an ingredient in some other food you are still eating?

7. Try not to get discouraged if you don't succeed instantly. Be prepared to modify your approach, and to

persist. Have a look at the section on **food exclusion** later in this chapter (pages 63 to 70) for more detailed help.

TYRAMINE AND OTHER AMINES IN FOOD

When food avoidance became a fashionable migraine treatment again about ten years ago, it was thought that a chemical called tyramine – which appears in the foods on the list in greater and smaller amounts – was the culprit. Tyramine and other naturally occurring amines in food, such as the 2-phenylethylamine in chocolate, are known to affect the way in which the blood vessels dilate and contract: they are called vasoactive for that reason.

Now, however, the role of tyramine has been questioned and even discounted by many experts. The foods can indeed precipitate an attack, but with the possible exception of those cheeses which contain high levels of tyramine, it is not clear which exact substance is the culprit. Tyramine just doesn't occur in sufficient quantity to be the problem. Some other ingredient, it is said, must be responsible.

Was it something I ate?

The most commonly named food triggers are **chocolate, cheese, citrus fruit**, and **fried food**.

Chocolate Cocoa contains a natural chemical substance called 2-phenylethylamine, an amine which has been thought to trigger migraine attacks. It also contains **caffeine**, another substance on the danger list.

Some researchers believe that it may not be the chocolate itself which is the trigger. This is not only because the amine levels in it are so low, but also because many migraineurs who report unusual hunger as a warning sign of an impending migraine, crave the sweetness of chocolate at that time. So, although it may seem as if it is the eating of chocolate that brought on the migraine, *wanting* the chocolate was a sign that the migraine syndrome had already swung into action, caused by some other trigger before the chocolate craving began.

However, it is definitely worth excluding chocolate from your diet completely, to see if your migraines are affected. You must cut out *all* chocolate and cocoa. No biscuits with a layer of it; no chocolate icing; no puddings with chocolate in them; no dusting of chocolate on your cappuccino . . .

If you are an unrepentant chocoholic, you can try carob-based chocolate preparations which are available in health food shops and don't contain any cocoa. And if you want to experiment with reintroduction, it's worth remembering that dark chocolate is often said to be worse than milk chocolate.

Cheesed off! Cheese is known to trigger migraines in some people, and the tyramine present in most sorts of cheese was, until recently, thought to be the culprit. Some people find that cooked cheese is a certain trigger, whilst raw cheese is safe. If the tyramine *is* the culprit, then **cottage cheese**, **quark**, **Philadelphia**, and **curd cheeses** should be fine, for they contain no detectable traces of tyramine. (The blue cheeses, and soft ripe cheeses in general, have the highest tyramine levels.)

Cheese may trigger migraine for some other reason. It may be that it delays the action of the stomach in absorbing food, and so it acts in the same way that eating too *little* food is known to do. But whatever the reason, it is a known danger area, to be treated with caution! If, however, you exclude cheese from your diet, do remember to compensate for the lost calcium, to help keep your bones strong.

Other dairy products, such as **milk** and **butter**, are also thought to trigger migraine in some people. This may be related to a question of food intolerance – allergies and intolerances to dairy products are not uncommon – or it could be caused by the high fat content of such foods. Fats are involved in the way vasoactive amines do their work, as well as in the metabolism of sugars. So you could try skimmed milk instead of full-cream or even half-fat milk – it's amazing how quickly your tastebuds adjust.

Citing citrus These contain another vasoactive amine called synephrine. There are higher levels of this in the skin of citrus fruit than in the flesh, and so **concentrated juices** are especially suspect because the skins are pulped and squeezed in its preparation, along with the flesh. If you want to exclude citrus fruits, check the ingredient lists on prepared foods for lemon and orange juices – and don't forget about **marmalade**!

A good British fry-up and other fatty foods Those vasoactive amines do their work best in the presence of fats, and so foods which contain high amounts of fats may trigger a migraine attack by increasing amine production and activity in your body.

However, it's also worth considering the whole picture: is it the fried foods themselves, or might it be the extra salt that you eat with a fish-and-chip supper? Are you eating processed foods which are then fried at home – and in that case, might it be certain flavouring or colouring additives, or preservatives, which are the real culprits?

One man discovered that the brand of tomato ketchup he used with fish and chips was to blame (it contained monosodium glutamate).

Food, migrainous food . . .

Other commonly mentioned potential food triggers include **bananas**, **pastry** and **pork**; **seafood** in general and **shellfish** in particular; and some vegetables as well – **onions** (fresh rather than dried ones) have been suggested, along with **pickles** and **chutneys** (it may be the vinegar that's the culprit, or a preservative, in these products). **Pickled herrings** contain a significant amount of tyramine, and so, I'm afraid, does **Marmite**.

Nuts are also frequently mentioned, and so are processed meats like **sausages** and **bacon**, because of the additives they contain.

Addled by additives

Many of the additives in prepared and packaged food are implicated in migraine. **Monosodium glutamate** (also known as MSG, or 621) is a 'flavour enhancer' that is used in food preparation – especially in Chinese restaurants, but it is also found in many convenience foods, in canned soups, and in instant foods such as the 'just add water' range of soups, noodles, and so on. You will have to search the labels of every packet you buy to exclude this additive from your diet. Some people are especially sensitive to it, and can recognise it instantly from the smell of the food.

Nitrates and **nitrites** dilate blood vessels, and so can affect people with a propensity for any sort of headache – including migraine. These are added to some prepared foods to 'enhance' their colour. Cured meats, such as most **sausages**, **hot dogs**, **bacon**, **salami**, and **ham**, usually contain nitrates and nitrites – so do some smoked and cured fish, like **kippers** and roll-mop **herrings**. High levels of **salt** have also been identified as a trigger by some migraine sufferers. Again, you will need to read every label with care if you want to exclude salt.

Food colourings such as **tartrazine** (E102), it is thought, are also potential migraine triggers. Because of the high levels of additives of various sorts in convenience foods and junk foods, it is a good idea to avoid them altogether if you suspect your migraines may have a food factor as a trigger.

Eating yourself allergic

There is no doubt that some people have found relief from migraine through treatment for food allergies, the most common being the exclusion of **wheat**, or **dairy products**, or **yeast** and **yeast-based foods**. Because it would be virtually impossible to run an acceptable scientific test to confirm or deny the truth of the successful results which are reported, it is very difficult for such treatments to gain positive medical attention, or scientific respectability. The subject of food allergy treatment is covered in more detail, on pages 66 to 70 and in Chapter Seven.

DRINKS THAT MAY GO TO YOUR HEAD

Red wine   This is an infamous culprit, but exactly why red wine can trigger migraine remains a bit of a mystery. The tyramine and phenylethylamine levels in red wine are very low, so they would be unlikely to precipitate an attack. However, it may be that the higher concentrations of the naturally occurring chemicals known as flavonoid phenols found in red wine (white wine has lower concentrations of these) are responsible.

Interestingly, the passage of time alters the composition of flavonoid phenols, and so the belief of many migraineurs that cheap red wine is more likely to bring on an attack than a more expensive vintage one may well be true. ('Pass the *premier cru*, please; my migraine threshold needs it.') Perhaps the phenols lose their propensity to trigger migraines over time – or perhaps, instead, cheap wine may contain additives which are themselves responsible. If you believe it may be the additives rather than the wine itself, you could try organic wine.

Other alcoholic drinks Other potential triggers are **port**, **brandy**, and **sherry**. Some people also have trouble with **beer**, and **whisky**. If you are concerned about the effects of alcohol on your migraines, it is probably best to avoid it completely for a month, and see if that has a beneficial effect.

Caffeine The caffeine in coffee and tea has also been cited as a migraine trigger, although it's also true that caffeine *withdrawal* is a common trigger (a delayed first cuppa of the day, for example). If you think caffeine may be a problem for you, it is worth trying decaffeinated coffee and caffeine-free tea instead of the 'real things'. The tea recommended to me, which I found delicious in its own right, is called **Rooibosch tea** (or, sometimes, **Eleven O'Clock tea**). You may find some of the herbal teas available an agreeable alternative to your usual brew. There are even some, like **Red Zinger**, specially formulated as a pick-you-up, so you needn't fear that the zip you look forward to each morning will necessarily be missing!

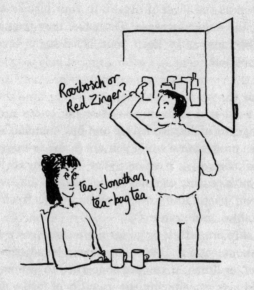

Again, the additives in tea and coffee might be a trigger, and you may want to try organic coffee and tea.

You should also remember that **Coca-Cola, Pepsi-Cola**, and other cola drinks contain caffeine.

DIETS CAN BE A HEADACHE

Just as some foods can trigger migraine, so too can the lack of food. Skipping or delaying meals, or not eating meals at regular times, can trigger migraine attacks as well, because a fall in blood-sugar levels triggers off a chain-effect. A sudden rise in blood sugar – when you eat

61

sugary food, for example – will be followed by an equally sudden drop as the level of insulin in your blood rises to cope with the sugar increase. That, too, may trigger an attack. The ideal is to keep your blood-sugar level as stable as possible.

Weight for it

This means that it is even less desirable to try a crash diet, or any sort of 'lettuce leaves and half-a-melon' quick weight-loss programme when you are prone to migraine, than it is normally. Keeping your blood-sugar levels steady involves eating complex carbohydrates (like whole-wheat bread, pasta, and brown rice) as well as fresh fruit and vegetables, and proteins.

Do not skip breakfast, or go for more than five waking hours without eating. Don't just have a sandwich or a plain salad for lunch. If you are concerned to lose weight, you should look at reducing the *quantity* of food you eat; try a Weight Watchers approach, and go for 'slow-but-steady' methods. (That won't just be good for your migraine, either: weight lost slowly will be more likely to stay off.)

Women who suffer from premenstrual migraines should be especially careful to maintain their blood-sugar levels during the danger period. A snack every three hours may well help, as long as it's not a chocolate or sugary one, which just makes the blood-sugar levels fluctuate wildly. Keeping them established and main-tained at a steady level is the aim. Try a piece of fruit instead of a chocolate bar, or a wholewheat crispbread or a sugar-free oatcake with a low-sugar jam or spread.

Some people whose migraines always begin in the morning have found a late-night snack to be an excellent way of avoiding attacks. Carol keeps a packet of oatcakes in a tin beside her bed, so she can have a couple whilst she's listening to *Book At Bedtime*. She might also have an extra oatcake if she wakes up during the night. 'I have an early dinner with my kids,' she explained, 'and when I heard about the blood-sugar theory, I realised that I went a long time between dinner and breakfast. And it worked!'

FOOD EXCLUSION

If you suspect that a particular food, or group of foods, may be the cause of your migraines (and keeping a diary may help you to pinpoint the culprits – see Chapter Five), then you will want to exclude them altogether from your diet. There are different sorts of food exclusion diets – and none of them ought to be tried without talking first to your GP.

You should always bear in mind that any food exclusion diet will have effects other than the one you intend – as well, with luck, as the one you do intend! In other words, there will be side-effects of some sort, for which you should be prepared. The effects are likely to make themselves felt at all levels, whether the exclusion is a simple one with just one identified element, or whether you are attempting a more complicated regime.

No food, or food too late?

Before you decide that a specific food, or group of foods, is the culprit, do spend some time trying to work out if a *lack* of food is really to blame – as it is for many migraineurs. Few people consider this as a potential problem, partly because it can be hard to spot. In the crisis of a delayed plane journey, for instance, you might be more likely to name the anxiety and annoyance as a stressful potential trigger. But the delay will also involve a much longer-than-usual interval between meals, and that's a likely trigger, too. So tracking the times at which you eat is well worth the effort.

The commonsense approach

No one wants to be a food faddist, unable to eat even the simplest of meals with friends without first embarking on an anxiously detailed conversation about ingredients and additives. It's bad enough having migraines, you may well think – I don't want to add a food problem to my social life! But sometimes, a commonsense approach will be all you need, and a special diet might not be necessary at all.

The first thing is to commit – to memory or to paper – the list of *likely* migraine trigger substances. And the second is to take a careful look at what you regularly eat. It may be something very simple, even very obvious (once you've spotted it!) that's causing the trouble. Once you've eliminated it, you may well have no further trouble from food.

So take some time to think, and to read the labels on *all* prepared foods. You may need to become familiar with the 'E' numbers used in the lists of ingredients (see the further reading list at the back of this book for help). Some people find that they have to give up all pre-packaged, convenience and take-away foods from their lives in desperation; you may be more fortunate. Only common sense will tell.

A simple exclusion diet

If you decide that **caffeine** may be the trigger for your migraines, you will probably decide to exclude all caffeine from your diet. So you will stop drinking coffee and tea; you will cut out Coca-Cola, Pepsi-Cola and other cola-type drinks; you will eliminate cocoa and hot-chocolate drinks. You will remember that caffeine is a potential ingredient in many compound pain-killers, and if you are taking Cafergot for migraine, you will need to consult your GP about the possibility of altering that medication too.

It is entirely likely that you will, within a few days of cutting out caffeine, have a very bad headache. You may feel shaky and nauseous; you may feel very irritable; you may have problems sleeping. These symptoms will disappear if you persist; they should vanish within a week of cutting out caffeine, and it will probably take less time than that.

Once that initial unpleasant hurdle is out of the way, you can begin to evaluate the positive effects of cutting out caffeine: on your life, and on your pattern of migraine attacks. Four weeks is the usual recommended test period for excluding something from your diet, and if your migraine attacks come frequently, that should be enough time. But if your attacks come every three or four weeks, you will have to exclude the caffeine for six to eight weeks; if they come less frequently than that, then the exclusion test period will have to be longer still.

If your attacks stop, or if they improve significantly, you will probably decide that the caffeine *was* responsible – and take no further action. If they don't, you'll need to try again with something else.

In order to 'prove' the caffeine's effect in an acceptably scientific way, it would have to be reintroduced into your diet, without your knowing for sure that it had, and its effects would have to be monitored. Personally, I think life's too short to play games like this with yourself, and if you've eliminated migraine, you'll be much too busy catching up with lost time to try double-blind experiments on your diet!

Of course, you might *want* to reintroduce the caffeine anyway – cautiously, in order to find out whether something you particularly like, perhaps something with relatively low caffeine levels, would be safe to take. Or you may have found that this particular exclusion has made no apparent difference. Don't be down-hearted. You *have* gained some knowledge; you *can* cross out one possible trigger – and you can continue the search.

An exclusion diet, properly conducted, is quite invasive enough an idea for most migraineurs. It may well be as much as you want to try, in the way of food-exclusion. But if your migraine attacks are very severe, or if you suspect that migraine is only one of the ways in which your body is 'trying to tell you something' about the food you eat and the way you live, then you might want to consider an elimination diet.

An elimination diet
An elimination diet is related to the theory of **food allergy** and **food intolerance**. It is a programme of eating which first eliminates all but a few 'control' foods, and then systematically reintroduces other foods and food groups. This is done in order first to identify, and then to neutralise, the culprit food or foods.

Supporters of a full-scale elimination diet argue that just excluding one food at a time won't do the trick – because your migraines may be related to more than one substance. You must cut out *all* suspect foods at once, to give you a response-free period. Once all the symptoms have disappeared, the foods are then reintroduced one at a time, to discover which ones produce the migraine. (*The migraine revolution* by Dr John Mansfield, published by Thorsons, is a straightforward guide to these ideas.)

An elimination diet is a diagnostic process, not a treatment in itself. So it isn't any good doing it half-heartedly, or coming off it for a day or two and then going back on it – you won't find out what you need to know. And you can't attempt it whilst also maintaining an active social life. You would also need to have at least a three-week period free from all social engagements, and in addition you will probably need the first week to be one in which no other demands are made on your time, energy, and concentration. This is a serious undertaking, and one which you shouldn't try without your doctor's knowledge – and preferably also their support.

The 'classic' exclusion diet confines your food intake to **twelve low-risk foods** – those which are least likely to cause an allergic reaction of any kind. The twelve foods are lamb, pears, cod, trout, plaice, carrots, courgettes, avocado pears, runner beans, parsnips, swedes and turnips. (The list was devised in the United States where people traditionally eat less lamb than in Britain. Since the twelve should also be foods which you eat uncommonly, the lamb is sometimes omitted, or changed to turkey, in Britain.)

All twelve foods should be purchased from **organic sources** if at all possible, to avoid the danger of a reaction from sprayed chemicals, and to avoid the possibility of other additives such as growth promoters. If you would normally eat any of the twelve foods on a regular basis – say, more than once every three or four days – then that, too, will have to be eliminated, just in case it is the culprit.

No **butter** or **cooking oil** can be used. Only **bottled spring water** can be drunk. All medications must be stopped (another reason why you *must* consult your doctor before you start) because many prescription medicines contain common food allergens such as filling agents, binders or sweeteners.

Corn, for example, is not only a common food as far as allergy and intolerance is concerned; it is also an extraordinarily commonly used additive in other foods. It appears as corn oil in almost all canned foods, in mayonnaise and salad dressings, and in many puddings. As corn syrup it is used in the production of ice cream, soft drinks, and processed meats, soups and sauces. **Corn starch** is used in almost all packaged food: in baby foods, in jams and pickles, in salt and sugar, and in dehydrated foods. It is the universal 'carrier' for pills, toothpaste and cosmetics. Insecticides often contain corn oil, so you're likely to get residues of that on fruit and vegetables, as well as the insect-killing chemicals. You will be hard pushed to avoid it.

For most of us – thankfully – such a programme is probably unnecessary. However, you needn't necessarily be deterred by the complications of the 'classic' programme. There are different sorts of elimination diet, ranging from a five-day fast through to an exclusion of just the most commonly offending foods, such as wheat and other cereals, dairy products, and eggs. No one should try a fast unsupervised – and especially not a migraineur! But there are other less stringent diets that you can try without danger.

For example, in *The complete guide to food allergy and intolerance* published by Bloomsbury, Dr Jonathan Brostoff recommends a three-stage elimination diet that begins

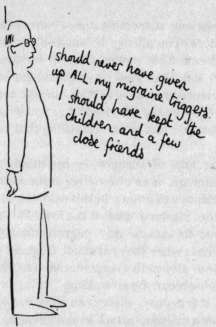

I should never have given up ALL my migraine triggers. I should have kept the children and a few close friends

with a one-month healthy eating programme. This excludes foods and drinks which have a drug-like action on your body, as well as sugary and processed foods. Some people find their migraines disappear during this phase, and so they have no need to continue. Stage two is a simplified elimination diet which excludes only the most commonly offending foods – and most migraineurs whose attacks have not disappeared in stage one, will find relief here. If they do not, then – and only then – is a more drastic treatment considered, involving either a 'few food' or a 'rare food' diet.

Masked allergies
It is possible to eat a particular food – especially every day, or on a regular basis – and to become allergic to the

food without suspecting it as a cause of the symptoms it produces. The allergy is 'masked' by the continuity of the doses. This means that if, for some reason, you *didn't* eat that food on a particular day, you would experience the same sort of allergic reaction (because your body *lacked* that food) that you would expect to get because you *had* eaten something that you were allergic to.

This line of thought is potentially interesting for migraineurs, as an alternative explanation of why fasting can induce a migraine. In this case, the sufferer is missing the next masking 'dose' of the food. The 'masking' theory is used to explain why migraineurs often have fewer migraines when they eat small, frequent meals – and it is also an alternative explanation for the frequency of migraine occurring on waking.

So, it is argued, allergy can work in two ways. You can trigger a migraine attack by not following your usual diet, or by eating a food which you only consume intermittently (say, less than once every five days). This is known as a reintroduction response.

If you want to know more about this subject, *The complete guide to food allergy and intolerance* by Dr Jonathan Brostoff is again a useful reference. And look at the section on clinical ecology in Chapter Seven.

Food combining diet

The Hay food combining diet has been around for almost sixty years, but it is only recently that it has gained attention as a possible relief for migraine sufferers. It may very well be worth a try for you.

There are five basic guidelines to be followed. Carbo-hydrates (sugars and starches) must not be eaten at the same meal as proteins and acid fruits. Vegetables, salads and fruits should make up the major part of your food intake. Proteins, starches and fats should, in contrast, be eaten in small quantities. No processed foods should be eaten – and that includes foods such as margarine as well as white flour and sugar. And finally, an interval of at least four hours should elapse between meals of different character – for example, between a carbohydrate-based meal, and a protein-based meal.

The cardinal rule is to avoid eating proteins and carbohydrates at the same meal, which means – just as an example – no sandwiches, flans or salads with a meat, cheese or egg filling. Fruit is divided into two groups: those which can be eaten at a protein meal, such as oranges and grapes; and those which can be eaten at a carbohydrate meal, such as bananas and dates. At first it can be hard to get used to the idea of food combining. The best book I've seen on the subject, however, has recipe and menu suggestions to try, and once you have got the hang of it, it's quite easy to remember. (The book is *Food Combining for Health; a new look at the Hay system* by Doris Grant and Jean Joice, published by Thorsons.)

Exactly why this diet should alleviate migraine is unclear. Perhaps its success is related to regularising mealtimes, or to avoiding processed foods. If you do want to try it, remember to be careful, while you are getting used to such a diet, that you don't skip a meal just because you can't work out the protein/carbohydrate balance. Give yourself time – and leeway – to begin with, and don't run the risk of low blood-sugar problems instead.

HORMONES AND MIGRAINE

Two sorts of migraine are linked to female hormone levels, and are common against women: **menstrual**, and **menstrually related**, migraine. Both of these are related to the changing levels of oestrogen, and progesterone, during the menstrual cycle.

Menstrual migraines

These tend to occur regularly, and in some women they are a direct result of hormone changes during menstruation. The migraine attack begins at the same time – from one or two days before bleeding starts, or up to three days after the bleeding begins. Treatment with an oestrogen 'patch' or cream prescribed by your doctor can sometimes help this sort of migraine.

Menstrually related migraine

Menstrually related migraines may occur at the same time as menstrual migraines, but they also occur at other stages of the menstrual cycle. Women who have this sort of migraine commonly suffer from other menstrually related problems as well, such as fluid retention, breast tenderness, and period pains. Hormone treatment may be less beneficial for this group, but careful maintenance of blood-sugar levels, and treatment of pre-menstrual symptoms, is often a good self-help programme to try.

Migraines and the pill

Some women, unluckily, find that their migraines have been triggered by using a combined oestrogen/progestogen pill. Many of these women suffer from migraines of increased severity or frequency whilst using the pill – or find that a pattern of migraines is re-established, after being free of them for years.

If you suspect that your migraine attacks are related to your use of the pill, or if the pattern of the attacks you have alters while you are using the pill, you must consult your doctor, urgently.

It may be a warning of an impending stroke, and you would have to stop taking the pill immediately. (Another form of contraceptive – perhaps even a different pill formulation – can usually be found.)

Migraines, the menopause and hormone replacement therapy

Many women experience their first migraine attack around the time of their first period, and their last around the time of the menopause. Unfortunately, however, some women continue to experience migraine attacks into their sixties and seventies.

It is worth asking your doctor about **hormone replacement therapy**, because in some cases, HRT – especially the patch – can ease the severity of migraines, or even help you to get rid of them altogether. But it is also true that beginning a course of HRT can trigger a new cycle of migraine attacks, or make the ones you already experience worse instead of better. This often happens not when the oestrogen level drops, but when the progestogen kicks in. Again, however, relief may come with HRT patches (especially the sort that combine oestrogen and progestogen).

You will need to work with your doctor, or perhaps a

specialist gynaecologist, to try to adjust the levels of oestrogen and progestogen. Some **migraine clinics** (the City of London one, for example: see the list of useful addresses at the back of the book) have special expertise here, and may be able to help you work out a programme to meet your needs.

OTHER COMMON TRIGGERS

It isn't possible to list every conceivable trigger for migraine, but here are those most often mentioned by members of the British Migraine Association, members of the Leicester Migraine Self-Help Group, and other migraineurs I have interviewed. Dealing with everyday life whilst trying to avoid triggers can seem daunting, but many people have succeeded. Some of their ideas appear briefly here, but others are dealt with in more detail in Chapters Four and Five.

Sometimes a social event, a journey, or a particular task, might expose you to a host of potential environmental triggers. But you have to live your life, go shopping, make journeys, and visit friends. So the trick is to find ways of avoiding certain combinations, or of lessening their effect on you. Finding out what causes your problem is the first step.

No smoke without fire

Many people find that their migraines ease or disappear when they stop **smoking** – or when others around them do so. Other people find that their own smoking, or other people's cigar or cigarette smoke, can intensify an attack. Just being in a smoke-filled room can do it for some people. There may be a link with the known effects of smoking on blood vessels.

George is sure that giving up smoking had a lot to do with his success in battling migraine. 'But it probably wasn't the only thing that helped,' he added. 'I found giving up smoking very, very difficult, and so I started to go running a lot to distract myself. And I stopped drinking so much, and I moved from a big city to a small town so my life became simpler too. So for me, giving up smoking was part of a whole process of taking my life in hand. But I haven't had a cigarette *or* a migraine for almost twenty years!'

Other smells and atmospheric pollution

After cigarette smoke, the most commonly mentioned potential triggers for migraine include **perfume, paint fumes, formaldehyde** (which is used in fabric manufacture, air fresheners, home insulation products, chipboard, toothpaste, and shampoo), **varnishes**, and **tar**. Some people also have a problem with **dry-cleaning fluids**.

Even smells that would be thought pleasant ones in other circumstances can trigger migraine. Strong, heavy **perfumes** like Passion are the most often mentioned. Some migraineurs find that the perfumes sold by the Body Shop, and the endearingly eccentric Cosmetics To Go mail-order company, are perfectly safe, presumably because their chemical composition is different.

Hair-spray is often found to be troublesome, too, and it would be worth switching to a kinder or unperfumed product (Cosmetics To Go has a gel, and the Body Shop has gels and a pump-action spray) if you have that problem.

Paint smells are difficult to avoid if you want to engage in any DIY at home. Some people find that the **masks** which are sold in trade decorating outlets are helpful – and remember that silk finish paints might be less of a problem than gloss paints. Using a **negative ioniser** in the room in which you are working can help, and so does making sure that the room is properly ventilated. (Both are also worth trying if you have a problem with the formaldehyde used in the sorts of DIY products listed above.) Negative ionisers are available from big chemists or department stores, and DIY stores.

The smell of **petrol** is frequently mentioned as a migraine trigger – and it may even be the true factor in a car journey, rather than car travel itself. You can try plugging a negative ioniser into the cigarette lighter in your car (the plug-in sort are on sale in car-accessory shops, and large chemists such as Boots) to cut down on exhaust fumes. You should certainly get the fuel line in your car checked, if the smell of petrol is persistent.

THE LIGHT BRIGADE

Strong and bright light, and flashing lights, are a certain trigger for many migraineurs. **Computer monitor screens** are a common problem, although it may be the fixed, unblinking gaze or the rigid sitting position that's the real culprit. Strobe lighting in **discos**; **fluorescent lights** in shops and offices – especially if they flicker; and **cinemas** or even badly adjusted **television screens**, can also be triggers. **Headlight glare** while driving at night, and the effect of the constant sweep of motorway lights past the side of the car, or something similar, can precipitate an attack.

Sometimes strong **patterns** on material or wallpaper can also trigger a migraine. A close stripe on a shirt, or zig-zag lines, or a pattern of dots on material, can make certain clothes impossible to iron if you're susceptible!

Wearing **sunglasses** – even indoors – can bring relief for people whose migraines are triggered in this way. For people who need to wear corrective glasses in any case, Reactolite-type glass (which darkens in strong light and returns to colourless glass indoors) is a useful choice.

A research programme in Cambridge recently discovered that tinted spectacles (coloured yellow, green, or blue according to what was most agreeable to the individuals) could prevent migraine in those who were sensitive to glare.

Do get your television set checked, and adjusted if necessary, if watching programmes seems to be a trigger. Many who are troubled in this way find that it helps to watch the screen with a moderate light from other sources, and not just from the screen itself.

EXERCISE DISCRETION

If you are unfit and suddenly undertake violent physical exercise, you can expect some unpleasant results, migraine or no migraine!

Some normally fit and active migraineurs, however, find that their attacks can be triggered even by moderate physical exercise. This may be related to blood-sugar levels, and sometimes taking a glucose tablet both before and after the exercise, and eating some complex carbohydrate afterwards (a wholewheat sandwich is often the easiest), will completely avoid a migraine.

Fitness does seem to help people improve their migraine status, but it is best to stick to exercise which doesn't place a sudden strain on your system. The once-a-week hard game of tennis or squash is not a good idea for migraineurs; swimming, brisk walking, or a gradually building work-out programme, would be less likely to cause problems.

I WORRY ABOUT MY ANXIETY LEVELS

Of all potential triggers likely to cause problems in the day-to-day realities of life, **stress** levels, and **anxiety**, are the biggest of all culprits which migraineurs must confront – and conquer.

Weekend migraines

It's generally thought that the pattern of attacks which leads to weekend migraines is related to contrasting patterns of stress: work during the week is filled with situations of tension and demand, and then – yippee! It's the weekend! You can relax for a while before you gird yourself for the following week's problems.

But perhaps relaxing is the last thing you're good at doing? Or perhaps your way of relaxing brings extra stress and strain on your body, or your mind – or both? Maybe you lie in bed on Saturday or Sunday morning, delaying or skipping breakfast, and thus playing havoc with your blood-sugar levels? Perhaps cutting into the vicious pattern of the week's work is a problem in itself, and you need to look at more positive ways of approaching your life as a whole, rather than in separate compartments of conflicting needs.

If weekends can be stressful, going away on **holiday** is ironically even more likely to bring on migraines. The stress and tension of getting ready and organised may seem to outweigh the pleasure of escape (or, perhaps, may add to feelings of guilt and anxiety about escaping from problems for a time).

The key to this is to make decisions for yourself about the stress, and about your responses to it. Once it's identified, you can find responses which are more positive for you, and which cut down on stress and anxiety levels.

Talk to someone else about these ideas – someone who knows you well. You may be surprised by their understanding and sympathy. Then look at the relaxation techniques suggested in Chapters Five and Seven, and choose one that appeals to you. At the first sign of a headache, or a particular stress trigger – as soon as you notice one of the 'four A-factors': (Anger, Anxiety, Aggravation or Annoyance), you can learn to swing into action with a simple remedy to slow down your responses.

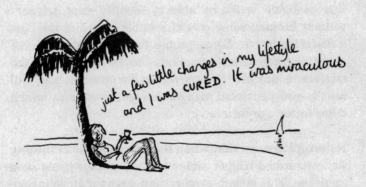

just a few little changes in my lifestyle and I was CURED. It was miraculous

A look at your life-style

By this stage of the book, you may be feeling as though the whole of life can be one big trigger factor! And if your life is packed with tensions, stresses, and anxieties, you may be well advised to take a long, hard look at your life-style. Maybe your migraines aren't an enemy at all; maybe in this case they're a friend, trying to tell you something important about what your system can and cannot stand.

Look at it this way. Life is not a rehearsal – this is *it*. It's up to you to make the most of it in the ways which matter to you. Some solutions are extreme – like changing your job, or the habits of a lifetime. Others are more gradual –like choosing something which you truly enjoy, and making time for it, and so also for yourself.

Consider them all, and choose the option that makes sense for *you*.

THE MIGRAINE MONITOR

You probably won't be able to identify your triggers without keeping some sort of reliable record of the patterns of your life. Some people find that filling in the migraine trigger chart is enough: they're lucky to find the triggers so quickly. Others persist for months, and still aren't sure just what trigger is combining with which other factor – or factors.

It doesn't always rain when there are clouds in the sky
An established trigger factor will not always bring on a migraine. This is both a relief, and a potential confusion. And it's also another good reason to keep a record that

covers a good chunk of time, and that's as full of information as possible. If you have enough evidence, you'll be more likely to name the clouds, whether or not they make rain every time they appear!

You need to find a way to record the basic information – a way that will work for you. If you do that accurately between one attack and the next, you will have an excellent chance of assessing the range of factors which trigger attacks for you.

There are lots of ways to keep such a record; three good ones are suggested in Chapter Five.

USEFUL ADDRESSES
Cosmetics To Go: telephone on 0800 373 366. From outside Britain, use the international dialling code plus 202 686666.

CHAPTER 4

Survival Techniques

Dealing with migraine is a process of discovery. When you are trying to defeat such a slippery customer as migraine, you need to develop some short-term strategies for coping, as well as some long-term solutions to fight it with.

This chapter is all about short-term strategies (long-term solutions come next, in Chapter Five). You will probably have developed some strategies for yourself, of course, but finding out about the methods that other people use to minimise the effects can help you to improve, extend, and adapt your own ideas.

Family support

The support and understanding of those you love, and those you work for, can be crucial. Many migraineurs feel that their family and friends don't really understand much about the condition. They may be sympathetic, but because migraine can be alarming to watch, they may also need reassurance about your condition at a time when you're least able to offer anything to anyone. They may rush to comfort and hold your hand, when all you want is to be left alone in the dark. They may offer good advice or treatments of various kinds, which may well be the very opposite of what you sense you really need. Or they may express irritation at your attempts to avoid an attack, or impatience with your techniques for dealing with one when it arrives.

'Not another headache?'
The understanding, even tolerance, of those you work for – and your colleagues at work – is also very important. One woman to whom I spoke is very fortunate: her immediate boss is also a migraineur, and so a sympathetic and interested response comes with the job!

Others are not so lucky. 'It isn't so much what's said,' pointed out one woman, 'it's more what is so obviously thought, but left *unsaid*. There can be a world of sarcastic innuendo in a phrase like, "Oh dear, not another headache?" '

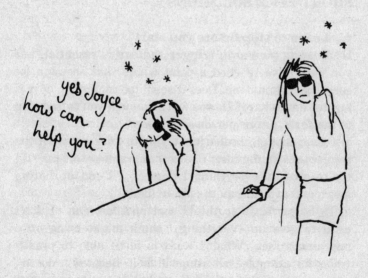

You might consider asking for a private word with your boss or colleague, if you find their attitude unhelpful or even hostile. You'll need to be patient and polite, and to marshal your facts in advance, so consider asking a sympathetic friend to come along. Don't just air the problems of migraine – make sure you emphasise the solutions you are trying to achieve. If you can involve their interest and engage them in the problem, you'll not only get a more positive response, but you may also get some help.

There is a section at the end of this chapter especially for your family, friends and work colleagues to read. Give it to them before your next migraine strikes, and help them to understand your condition and your needs.

SHORT-TERM SOLUTIONS

1.   Learn to stop before you start

Discovering your own **trigger factors** is essential, but you may have reached a point where that seems a lot easier said than done. Does it seem too confusing, or is it just too damn hard? Do you feel as though you're 'fighting in the dark', as one person said to me?

'I have enough trouble just trying to work out what the triggers are, in my case,' one new migraineur told me. 'If I try to give up everything I suspect, I'll end up hating meals and avoiding all the fun in life.'

'To be perfectly truthful,' said another man, 'I don't *want* to give up everything I think might bring on a migraine attack. What I want is to be able to predict when, for example, red wine will do it. Because it doesn't *always* trigger a migraine. It would be great to be able to know when it would and when it wouldn't.'

'When I first got the list of tyramine-containing foods, I was free of migraine for about six months,' Fiona told me. 'But I found all that constant attention to what to eat and what not to eat made me very uneasy. I didn't want to know about being ill on such a constant level of attention. I just want to get on with life, really.'

'I don't know what I *can* do,' said another. 'I think I just have to put up with it.'

Do you recognise any of those comments in your own response to migraine?

THE CHOICE IS YOURS

Sometimes we are our own worst enemies, and we allow ourselves to play complicated mind-tricks and games. We make choices we think we really ought *not* to have made – and so we pretend that we didn't really make them, or that they weren't really choices. In this respect, migraineurs are no different from other human beings!

The truth is, you *don't* have to put up with migraine – but you can choose to do so, if you want to. There are lots of things to try, and just deciding to try them puts *you* in control, rather than the migraine. From my own experience, I believe you'll feel better if you have a go.

But *you* must make the choice. You can choose between having migraine attacks, and working out how to manage them. It may be that your migraine attacks are infrequent, and the pain, though unpleasant, is endurable. Perhaps, then, you'd rather have them than go through the process of working out how to stop them. That's fine – if you're sure you won't regret giving up the chance to get rid of them completely.

FEELING A FAILURE

But perhaps you have begun work on managing your migraines, and have so far not succeeded? Are you feeling depressed because your efforts haven't yet identified anything helpful? Worse still, perhaps you have found a likely trigger factor but even with the exclusions, your migraines haven't gone away. Obviously, there's something else that still needs to be tackled.

No one said it would be easy. You're very lucky if your first few tries at identifying and excluding a potential trigger are successful. It isn't easy at all – but it *is* worth persisting. It all boils down, at times like this, to working on your attitude as well as on your migraines. One step at a time; one thing at a time. The next step may be the successful one. After all, you have nothing to lose from a positive attitude – except, of course, your migraines! And you are not alone – neither in your bouts of despondency, nor in your search for a personal cure.

2. Predicting the problems

You have won half the battle if you can think ahead and, like a good girl guide, be prepared.

WHEN THE UNEXPECTED HAPPENS

If you are one of those who can control the triggers pretty well when you're at home, but have a lot of trouble with migraine when you're away from home, don't despair. It can be done: it just takes a bit of pre-planning.

Plan for the unexpected to happen, and be prepared for things to go wrong. That way, if they do, *you* won't make the situation worse through your anxiety; instead, you'll feel in control and able to cope, which is by far the most helpful way to approach any difficulty.

GOING PLACES

Suppose that you have to travel to another city, perhaps for a business meeting. There's plenty of time for the journey, and for you to collect your thoughts on the way, so stress shouldn't be a problem. But then the train is late or cancelled, and you have to make quick alternative arrangements that throw you into a flurry of mental readjustments. You catch another train, and readjust as best you can – but the replacement train doesn't have a buffet car; you have to sit in the bright sunlight all the way; your adrenalin levels are up; and you're missing lunch.

If you often make long-distance journeys for work, have a kit always packed and ready in your briefcase or your handbag. Always keep a supply of **emergency food** in it. A few mini-packs of sultanas and some oatcakes are a good idea, so that you can maintain your blood-sugar levels in an emergency. You can add some fresh fruit and a sandwich on the day itself, especially if it's a journey that could overlap a mealtime, or if you're unsure about meal arrangements at the other end. And include a small bottle of mineral water, or a small thermos of a hot drink or soup.

Having food with you not only means that you're maintaining your blood-sugar levels, but it also means that you don't have to rely on supplies of confectionery or snack food – all likely sources of additives of various sorts and so potential triggers in themselves.

GLARINGLY OBVIOUS

If bright light is a potential trigger for you, always keep a spare pair of **sunglasses** to hand. Some people find the wrap-around sort best, because they stop light catching them from the side: Polaroid Visions PL009 is one recommended brand. Another useful kind is designed to drop inside prescription glasses, and it includes side-pieces (in Britain, the brand name is Specsavers). If you have trouble tracking down the wrap-around kind, try sports shops which stock sunglasses worn for skiing.

PAIN-KILLERS ON CALL

Always have some **pain-killers** with you. Decant some of your usual brand into a small container (I use the plastic snap-top containers that photographic film is sold in), and that to your travel kit. The sort you can swallow without needing to dissolve them in water are best for journeys, of course, so if you usually take soluble ones, you could consider replacing them with the same brand or type in pill or capsule form. If you use a particular **anti-migraine drug**, have it with you. If it is available in syrup form, have that with you in preference (and then you won't need to worry about finding a liquid to take it with), again decanted into something suitable. (Chemists and department stores often stock small screw-top plastic containers you can use, or you could recycle plastic sample bottles of cosmetics.)

You can keep everything you may need in a small plastic bag, or a spare makeup purse, or inside one of those zipped containers that some airlines give away. Think about what you need *now*. Make a permanent list. Never leave home without the kit. Check the list through when you are packing, to make sure nothing needs replacing.

SOME FOR THE ROAD

Have a separate, permanent **car kit** always waiting in the glove compartment or pocket of the car (and remember to replenish it when you use up the stocks). Add a bottle of **mineral water** as well. If you know that you have trouble with petrol smells or exhaust fumes when you're driving on motorways or filling up at stations, keep a plug-in **ioniser** in your car kit, ready to go into the cigarette lighter before you drive away (see page 76). Consider, too, wearing a nose-and-mouth **mask** of the kind that cyclists wear in cities.

The problem of glare for car travellers can sometimes be dealt with by wearing a **sun hat**, or a hat with a brim floppy enough to stop light flickering in your eyes as you drive. Or you could take the advice of a member of the British Migraine Association, who bought a strip of the **tinted plastic** sold in car-accessory shops intended to minimise windscreen glare. He cut this to fit along the tops of the *side* windows, so making a light-diffuser for the driver and the driver's companion.

If by now you are enjoying the absurdity of imagining yourself driving along swathed in a floppy hat, wraparound sunglasses, and a face-mask – then yes, all this certainly does have its funny side. You may well look rather eccentric! But does that count as high as successfully avoiding a potential migraine trigger? Only you can say.

3. Take a deep breath

If you can cope with the physical effects of a stressful situation, you will help yourself prevent it from triggering a migraine.

You may not even realise how tense your body

generally is, even in situations when you consider yourself to be relatively at ease. Even when you are sitting comfortably at home, perhaps listening to family chat or to a television or radio programme, it's very unlikely that you are *truly* relaxed.

Your jaw muscles, for example, are very probably tense. Check that, right now, by stretching out your chin and neck, consciously tense the muscles of your jaw and face, and then, consciously, relax and let them go.

Were the muscles tense to start with? Lots of people are surprised how tense they really are – and how often that tension makes itself felt in daily life.

Try that exercise every time you remember: whenever you take a break from work, or look up from your desk, or start down another aisle in the supermarket. Flex your shoulders, too – you will probably find that they're a bit hunched and tense as well. You'll soon be able to consciously alter that tense state to a more relaxed one, in just a few seconds.

OWN UP TO BEING HUMAN!
When you are in a situation that makes you feel nervous, or tense, or upset, the first thing to do is to admit it's so. Don't pretend that you're an invincible superhuman – or, if you must, at least don't pretend it to yourself!

The second thing to do is to turn your usual, automatic reaction to stress into a more positive one. To do this, you need to develop some sort of inner conversation technique with yourself: a sort of monitoring, continuing dialogue which acknowledges the way you're feeling and responding, but which reminds the stressed self of other ways of coping.

Does that sound too silly to contemplate? Yet it's not

much different from many other ways in which we assess situations and come to terms with them, only this time it's private, and designed to reduce and to change certain bad habits into good ones. It's designed to avoid turning a potential stress trigger into a full-blown migraine attack. So it's worth a try.

BODY LANGUAGE

When you feel your jaw tightening, your pulse starting to increase, your mouth drying and your neck muscles seizing up – *stop*.

Say 'STOP THIS!' to yourself firmly, but kindly; you are taking control of yourself, but you don't have to turn into a headmistress.

If you're alone, you can say it out loud. If you're in company, you need to be able to hear the tone of voice you use in your head. Practise it now.

Then take a deep breath, and let it out slowly. *Feel* the breath escaping out, and away. Take another, and repeat that slow exhaling of breath.

Now say to yourself, out loud or in your head, whichever's appropriate: 'BREATHE IN PEACEFULNESS. BREATHE OUT TENSION.'

Every time you breathe in, think of calm, quiet, soothing things. Or just think of the word 'peaceful'.

Every time you breathe out, think about letting go of the tension and anxiety. Try visualising the tension – perhaps as tight little balls of knotted string, or screwed-up bits of paper, blowing away from you and dissolving in the air beyond you.

Do that ten times.

Then start the job again, taking it slowly, step by step.

It really helps, I promise.

4. Signs and portents

Learning to take notice of the migraine **warning signs** is a life-saver for many people; for others it remains an unconquerable mountain.

Some people have warning signs they can learn to recognise, while other people never know until they wake up with the edge of a headache. Sometimes it's easier for your family or friends to notice unusual alterations in your behaviour than it is for you. So ask them to help you, and look back at pages 21 to 22 for some more suggestions.

Next time you have a migraine attack, think back as comprehensively and as clearly as you can (you will probably have to wait until the attack is over to do this). What happened the day before? Were there any **feelings** you can identify, in retrospect, that might be attached to the start of a migraine? Did you feel unusually depressed or elated? Did you feel giggly for no good reason? Or especially talkative? Did you feel unusually **tired**, almost as though you were 'sickening for something', or did you feel as though it was especially hard to get your thoughts together, or your words into sentences?

And were there physical signs? Did you feel especially **hungry**? Did you suddenly crave a particular sort of food? Did you feel **bloated** or **uncomfortable**? Did you have any **digestive upsets** – maybe needing to pass urine more or less than normal, or perhaps being constipated?

This might all sound a bit like 'twenty-twenty hindsight' – easy enough to think of after the event, but impossible to identify at the time. But it just takes practice, and learning to be more aware of your own body and mind, and to 'tune in' to differences. You can only begin by thinking about it after the event – but you can learn to predict as well.

So start with thinking back after the event. Ask your family to help. If you do manage to identify a warning sign the evening before, act *immediately* to try to prevent a full-scale migraine attack from occurring. Take your migraine pills, or try the strategies listed below, or try out something you think will work. Learn to trust your own instincts; listen to your body. Ask *yourself* what will help, and follow your own advice, if you can. Put yourself in control of your own symptoms, and your own remedies.

HOME AND AWAY

If you are away from home

For many migraineurs, this is the central incapacitating dread of their lives: that a migraine attack will happen when they are away from home. Somehow, they will have to cope with explaining the problem to other people, trying to organise what they need to get through an attack, asking for the right support and isolation without being a burden or disrupting other people's pleasure (or work) too much – and all whilst actually experiencing the pain and dislocation of the attack. It is, indeed, a hellish scenario.

No wonder many migraineurs avoid travel, avoid holidays, choose (or are forced into) desk-bound jobs, and gain a reputation for being social recluses.

Some people dread having to explain that they have a migraine coming on, and no, it isn't just a headache, and yes, I feel sick and just need . . . No, thank you, I'd rather not have company/a hot water bottle/a phone call in half an hour to see if I'm better/a brisk walk/a cup of tea. I want a darkened room, I want no noise or conversation, and I want to be left to sleep it off.

If you don't want to explain, *don't*. If you'd rather tell a lie, then do so. Don't feel guilty, either – tell yourself you'll deal with all of that when you feel better. Right now you have to concentrate on only one thing: coping with the attack.

You can try saying simply that you feel sick and nauseous. Say as firmly as you can that you know what's wrong, and you know what will cure it. Don't try to go into details if you can't think straight or are feeling anxious and panicky; say what will get the best results, in the quickest time.

Suppose you have to attend something like a residential sales conference – a situation that many people experience in their working lives – and you worry that a migraine may strike. What can you do in advance?

Plan to take an anti-migraine kit with you – the kind described on pages 87 to 89, earlier in this chapter. Think ahead, list the things you know will help you both to avoid – and to endure – an attack, and make sure you have them with you.

Consider having a private word with your boss, or the conference organiser, or even the hotel manager, in advance. You might prefer not to do that – but do at least think about whether that would help. What would you want to establish, ahead of time? How could that help? If it would, how could you phrase it so as to put yourself in a positive light, and avoid the chance of sounding either like a neurotic worry-wart, or a self-centred hypochondriac?

If it can be done, or if it's worth a try, then you might want to give it a chance.

Know what you will say and do, if an attack does begin. Work it out ahead of time. Have a strategy you can put into action right away. Keep all this to yourself, if you prefer. It feels powerful just knowing in advance that you can cope; you don't have to tell anyone else, unless you want to.

Don't hang around

If you wake up with a headache away from home, weigh up the consequences of trying to kill off the attack quickly, and the consequences of *not* doing so.

If you take your regular pain-killer immediately, take the phone off the hook, hang out the 'Do Not Disturb' notice, draw the curtains tightly, pull the covers over your head, and go back to sleep – then you may well avoid a fully fledged attack. You may wake up a few hours later and find you have managed to prevent the worst of the attack from happening.

In most cases, that's wonderful. But if your presentation is supposed to happen at 9.00 a.m., you may decide that it would be better not to cancel or move it. So you will have to endure the consequences.

You may also decide that you'd rather endure a full migraine than the aftermath of a half-avoided attack. For some people, that makes sense – and so they spend most of their detective energy tracking down and dealing with eliminating triggers, rather than on identifying early warning signs.

That's not silly; that's intelligent decision-making, for them. And for me, it rings a familiar bell.

My migraine attacks sometimes last for three days. They're not as bad as some people's; and they're worse than others'. I hate them, and I do what I can to avoid them – and now, that's almost always successful. But sometimes it's not.

When one threatens, I have to work out what's better for me in the circumstances. Should I try to knock it on the head immediately, and so probably lose only that day's working time? Or should I grit my teeth and soldier on with the job that's critical that day? Then the migraine *will* hit – with luck, not until after I've got the work done – and I'll lose the next day or two instead.

If I take my migraine pills right away and retreat to bed, the headache won't get worse, but I'm likely to suffer a great tiredness and loss of energy for *more* than three days, in consequence. So I shall be able to continue to function – but at a much less effective level.

So, which is the better choice? It depends on the circumstances. I have always chosen, so far, to knock the attack on the head, and hope that the tiredness and lethargy won't last for as long as before. But if you have something you simply must do that morning, and you *can't* hide away in order to cure it, then your decision might be different.

One leading ballerina to whom I spoke managed to perform for years, through the most appalling migraines. She would retch and vomit in the wings, and then return to the stage impeccably on cue, and dance with all her usual musicality and technical skill. She used, I think, a combination of an exceptionally strong will and the years of rigorous training to see her through these most difficult of circumstances – and no audience ever guessed there was a problem, or was ever disappointed by her performances.

I try to remember her courage when I doubt my own ability to get through the next few minutes, or the next few hours, of my own far less invasive symptoms.

QUICK REMEDIES TO TRY IN AN EMERGENCY

A strong cup of coffee or tea
If you are avoiding caffeine as a potential trigger, this is not a good strategy to try. But if you need to keep yourself together and functioning for just an hour or so, caffeine can help you to do so.

Two or three glasses of fizzy mineral water
I suggest *fizzy* water because it can help in dealing with nausea (and so can a sweet fizzy drink like Coca-Cola, but treat that with caution because of its caffeine, too). Lemonade or Lucozade might also work. Some people have found that drinking lots of water (six to eight glasses a day) really helps when their migraine resistance feels dangerously low.

A cup of tea and a biscuit
Try whatever seems right to you – don't force yourself to eat something if that idea cries out a warning of worse effects! But in an emergency, weak sweet tea (try honey rather than sugar), and a dry biscuit, can get you through. And so, of course, can sitting down in peace and quiet to enjoy the snack.

A cup of herbal tea

Try out different sorts before an attack strikes, so that you can decide in advance which may help. **Camomile** may make you feel relaxed and dozy and so help you to sleep off the attack; **peppermint** may help to soothe and settle a nauseous stomach; **Red Zinger** may give you enough of a lift to carry you through.

Food of some sort

Many migraineurs find the idea of food impossible the moment an attack threatens, but for others, eating something can help to stave off – or to mitigate – the effects. I've read about a number of apparent oddities which people have found to be life-savers: honey sandwiches; a baked potato; chicken soup. If you think food may help, then try your own particular comfort remedy. If you are revolted by the thought, don't force yourself.

Breathing into a paper bag

This old remedy really works for some people. As soon as the first signs of an attack begin to show themselves, you take an ordinary paper bag, blow into it to expand it, and then take five or six breaths with your mouth pressed to the opening. Then take the bag away and breathe normally again. You can repeat the treatment three or four times.

This works by increasing the levels of carbon dioxide in your bloodstream, and so dilating the blood vessels in your head. If it is going to work for you, it will probably only do so at the onset of an attack.

A hot shower

One migraineur I know manages to push her migraines

away, when they arrive first thing in the morning, by washing her hair and using extra-hot water to do it. Another recommends a long hot shower followed by a very quick cold rinse. Both of these remedies probably work by relaxing muscle tension, so they need to be put into practice as quickly as possible.

Blow it away

And before you think I have completely lost my marbles with *this* suggestion, I can only defend myself by saying that not only have several people I've talked to sworn by this as a method, but I've also found an historical connection for it!

In the eighteenth and nineteenth centuries, the taking of snuff was sometimes recommended for migraine attacks, because it was thought that a really big sneeze or two would do the trick. I've met two people who say that sneezing (without the snuff, I hasten to add) works for them, and another who says that if she blows her nose hard at the first signs of a migraine headache, she manages to get rid of it. Maybe it's related to blood-pressure levels; coughing and sneezing are a very common way of raising these inside your head.

PLEASE YOURSELF

Experience will teach you what comforts you during a migraine attack: what you crave, and what you dread.

Attending to your own needs is an essential step towards self help in a migraine attack. Do *not* do what other people think you should, unless it makes sense to you too. Do *not* try to please other people. Try to please yourself, and relieve the symptoms with as little fuss and as much success as you can manage.

A dark and quiet place

If you can't manage this exactly as you wish when you are away from home, you will have to improvise. I have in my time used an **airline sleeper mask** to cut out light (it was surprisingly effective; you might keep one in your kit), and **ear-plugs** to mask day-time sounds. That was less effective, but another brand of ear-plug might work better.

Hot- and cold-packs

Many migraineurs make themselves feel more comfortable by the application of extremes of temperature. For some, only **ice-packs** will do; for others, the very *thought* of a **hot water bottle** pressed against the side of their head is enormously comforting.

Some people find that clutching an ice-pack or a hot-pack to their head, neck or stomach does the trick. They may find relief from using a **'cold hat'** – a plastic device rather like a shower cap that you can keep in the freezer, and wear at the first sign of a headache. (Some mail-order companies sell these, as do some department stores.)

You will most certainly look pretty silly in it, but by this stage of an attack, you are very unlikely to care about that. Quite frankly, I'd stick my head in a teapot and sing 'Moon River' if I thought it would help.

If you find hot water bottles too bulky, you could try the special packs which are sold in chemists, or you can use the kind which keep food hot or cold by being either boiled in water or popped in the freezer. (One of these might need to be added to your emergency kit.)

Chemists also sell **hand-warmers** of various kinds, and these would make excellent sense for an emergency kit. You don't have to use them on your hands, of course; you could also tuck them inside your collar to relieve pain in your neck and shoulder muscles. You could also consider the gel-filled **eye packs** which are sold as a beauty treatment in chemists and department stores. The gel can be warmed or cooled, and retains its temperature pretty well.

In an emergency, an ice-pack can be created by a pack of frozen vegetables like peas (just don't eat the peas after they've thawed and hung around in bed with you for hours). And a face flannel wrung out in hot or cold water is a lot better than nothing.

Some people find that alternate applications of hot- and cold-packs is very helpful. Many sufferers find that they get very cold during an attack, and so need extra bed-clothes, or socks, or more than one hot water bottle (one for the feet, and perhaps another to soothe an upset stomach).

Nausea remedies

If you don't want to try one of the anti-nausea drugs, or if you can't take them for some reason (like pregnancy), you might find relief by using **sea-bands** on your wrists. These are natural remedies for travel sickness and nausea, which grip around your wrists and act on the pressure points there; most chemists stock them. Many migraineurs find them very useful.

Muscle tension

A lot of people find this a problem during a migraine attack. Muscle tension seems to increase, and to settle especially into your neck and shoulders, so that finding a comfortable position to ease the pain can be very difficult.

A **neck pillow** – one of those sausage-shaped supports sold by large department stores, specialist back shops, and some chemists – can be a real help here. Or try soothing the muscle pain with **Tiger Balm** or **Olbas oil**, or with **rosemary** or **lavender** oil (dilute these first if you buy essential oils). Olbas oil is a great help both in clearing the nasal congestion which accompanies a migraine for me, and also for easing the pain in my neck and shoulders. But do remember all these oils have very distinctive smells!

Your doctor might prescribe an **analgesic gel** that you could use. Ibugel, for example, is an ibuprofen-based gel which works well on muscle pain.

ACTING SPEEDILY

The one thing that counts above all when a migraine attack begins is to act with speed, and marshal your remedies against it. If you take pain-killers, take them right away; don't wait for the pain to get worse. If you take anti-nausea pills, or any medication with an anti-nausea element in it, then speed is of the very essence of its effectiveness. If you wait until later, your digestion may have slowed down in that classic migraine effect called **gastric stasis**, and any medication you take by mouth will be of little use to you.

And act quickly, too, with whatever other remedies you want to try out. Having an attack away from home is a frightening and lonely business, but it will be helped by your attitude towards it. Panic and misery will not help you to cope with the migraine. On the other hand, a positive approach to putting your strategies into action will really help you to feel as though you are in charge, doing the best you can.

Reading through the suggested self-help strategies in Chapter Five will also provide extra pointers about emergency action. Pressure points, relaxation techniques, self-hypnosis: these are all worth having up your sleeve for a crisis, as well as for any regular attacks you have at home.

GETTING HELP

There are several ways in which you can seek help for the present, as well as help for the future.

1. If you are away from home, in or near a city with an emergency migraine treatment centre, **professional help** could be a great relief. Look at the list of clinics at the back of this book to see if you could get help that way. I keep a copy of the British list in my emergency kit, just in case. I do know I'm not going to remember addresses in the middle of a migraine, but knowing that I have a list of emergency sources of help to hand is a comfort.

2. You really should have a discussion with your doctor about modern **drug treatments**. Many migraineurs have not talked to their GP for years, and have no idea of the range of drugs now available, nor of the effects of modern research on their condition.

I'm not saying that you have to take drugs, or that a modern 'miracle' drug is necessarily a better answer than the one you are already using. But knowledge is better than ignorance, and you may learn a lot from a straightforward consultation. Check the advice on pages 121 to 123 before you go, to make sure you are armed with as much information on your side of the desk as possible. It can make a big difference to the questions you ask, and to your doctor's responses.

3. Try to **help yourself**, as far as the stresses and strains of your working life are concerned. Try to spread the load of your work patterns as evenly as you can; pace yourself, and don't allow any absurdly unreasonable demands to take their toll, if you can possibly avoid it. Working frantically hard and then collapsing in a heap is a common migraine trigger. Smooth out the pattern as much as you can.

4. Learn techniques to deal with your own responses to stress, anxiety, and disappointment. Talk to a stress counsellor; try massage; look at the self-help strategies suggested in the following chapter. **Take yourself seriously.**

MIGRAINE IN CHILDREN

The only significant difference between migraine in childhood and in later life is that most children who suffer from migraine have accompanying attacks of abdominal pain. The same range of treatments available to adults are used for children, although aspirin should *not* be given to children, and any prescribed drug will be given in much smaller doses.

Several studies have shown that most childhood migraine can be successfully controlled or entirely avoided through a careful maintenance of blood-sugar levels. So **regular meals, late-night snacks**, and a good **breakfast**, are all worthwhile strategies to try.

If your child seems to be reporting the symptoms of

migraine, **medical advice** is an important first step to take; reassurance for both of you will help. And make sure the school understands the problems – and the potential triggers – so that they can help your child to avoid certain situations without fuss or anxiety. (If drugs are prescribed, too, make sure the school knows about their use.)

FAMILY AND FRIENDS: HOW TO BE HELPFUL

This is the section especially written for your family and friends to read. It contains some practical dos and don'ts, and some advice about helping.

Six things you can do
1. Empathise
Spend just a minute or two imagining a combination of a violent headache which throbs and lurches around when you move your head; uncontrollable vomiting and nausea; shivering and sweating at once; and a feeling of dislocation, despair and fear. That's how migraine feels, for hours or days at a time. Try to remember that, the next time arrangements have to be altered or cancelled because of a migraine attack.

2. Support
Be as supportive as you can about the sufferer's efforts to avoid a migraine. You may see the avoidance techniques as sheer awkwardness, and respond with irritation – but the sufferer is just trying to avoid the next attack. Your understanding can make all the difference to success or failure. After all, it's in your interests as well that the migraine is brought under control.

3. Help

Try to make social arrangements as flexible as you can, to avoid disappointment or elaborate rearrangements. No one has a migraine on purpose; the sufferer is not doing this to annoy you, or to get out of something. What's more, reducing the stressful anxiety involved in disappointing or annoying you will help prevent a migraine from striking.

4. Talk

Work out in advance what help would be welcomed during an attack, and what would simply increase the difficulties. Don't just do what you would like; *ask* before the attack hits what would be appreciated.

5. Encourage

Help the sufferer to identify the warning signs, or even the potential triggers, of an attack. It's often an outsider who is best placed to spot someone else's patterns of behaviour or of eating. You could provide the key to a solution.

6. Remember

Learn how best you can help, both during an attack and before it strikes. Then make sure that's what your response concentrates on, rather than on offering your own ideas.

Most migraineurs will be very grateful for any help on their behalf in sorting out any necessary arrangements and adjustments to the family time-table. You may be able to telephone to cancel appointments, take the children off somewhere so their noise won't be a disturbance, make sure the radio doesn't penetrate, and generally keep the household functioning. But do ask first!

Six things you should try to avoid
1. No offence
Don't take it personally. No one has a migraine attack to avoid your company – it just doesn't work that way! On the other hand, if you behave in a very unhelpful or difficult way, it may well be that the migraineur *will* want to avoid your company in the future!

2. No blame
Don't spend time making the migraineur feel guilty about the effects of their migraine. Maybe it *has* made you late, or made you miss out on something special, but letting them know that won't help anyone. Migraineurs spend too much of their time feeling guilty and anxious, and you shouldn't encourage that.

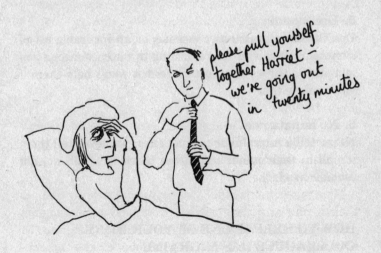

please pull yourself together Harriet – we're going out in twenty minutes

3. No interference

Don't offer help constantly during an attack, or hover at the bedroom door to offer advice and suggestions, unless you have specifically been asked to do so. Most migraineurs crave only to be left alone during an attack, though they'll probably welcome a basin and clean cloths during the vomiting phase.

4. No misunderstandings

Don't be cross or hurt if you don't get much sense out of the sufferer during a migraine attack. Many migraineurs can't think or talk coherently whilst an attack is in progress. It's another common side-effect, and once again it has nothing to do with you personally. It's not a criticism; it's just part of the whole syndrome of migraine.

5. Don't panic

Don't treat migraine as a disease, or an incurable set of symptoms. It can be very alarming to watch someone you love in the throes of an attack, but it won't help them if you panic, either.

6. No impatience

Never tell a migraineur to snap out of it; never tell them it's all in their mind; and *please* never say, 'Oh no, not *another* headache!'

HOW TO HELP IF ONE OF YOUR WORK COLLEAGUES HAS MIGRAINE

1. Try to help avoid migraines in the first place. The **environment** in which people work can play a critical

role in helping to reduce the frequency of migraine attacks, as well as the likely severity of them.

2. Is the **lighting** up to scratch? If there are fluorescent lights, it's very important to make sure they don't flicker: high-frequency fluorescent lights are better in that respect. Lights shouldn't shine directly into the face of anyone, whether they have migraine or not, but glare is a known trigger, and should be especially avoided.

3. **VDU screens** are a problem area for many people. Lights shouldn't be allowed to reflect off the VDU monitor or the keyboard. If the background can be adjusted (and it often can), then choose a black background with white or green characters against it, rather than black characters on a white background.

EC regulations state that VDU workers are entitled to have an anti-glare screen fitted to their monitors. This may help prevent migraines, but it's likely that seating and lighting will play an equally important part. If your colleague is hunched forward peering at the screen or squinting against a glaring light, the muscle tension alone can trigger a migraine.

4. Encourage regular **breaks** from work. People work better if they have a few minutes' break from work every hour. VDU users should rest their eyes from the screen every ten minutes or so. **Fresh air** and **noise reduction** are also important.

5. If a migraine strikes, then the following points will help deal with it:

★ Encourage your colleague to keep an emergency kit at work, so that medication is on hand.

★ Try to arrange for a quiet, dark place to be available so that people can rest at work if necessary.

★ Offer a lift home if your colleague is too ill to drive, or ensure that a lift is available to them.

★ Don't allow others to mock or 'bad mouth' your colleague's problems behind their back. You wouldn't do that with another illness, would you?

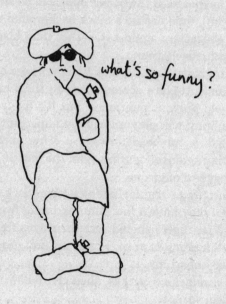

what's so funny?

CHAPTER 5

How Can You Stop Them?

PAST, PRESENT AND FUTURE

The first step towards tackling long-term management or prevention of migraine is to gather the evidence. You need as much evidence about your attacks as you can possibly assemble, and so you will need to keep a full and accurate record, not just of the attacks themselves, but of your life – what happens, and how you feel about it.

Dear Diary

If you are already a diarist, this will be familiar territory for you. If you are not, and you are unaccustomed to the routine of daily record-keeping, it may feel rather a burden until you get into the swing of it. Maybe even the idea of keeping a migraine diary fills you with gloom. Why should you do it? Will it really help?

Keeping a record *will* help in several ways – and in unexpected ones, as well as the obvious. The information is the essential part, but the process of recording it can also be a very positive one.

'I found that writing up my diary each day helped me *not* to dwell on my migraines,' explained one migraineur I talked to. 'It only took me a few minutes each day, and then I could put it *and* my anxieties aside for the rest of the day. A bit like therapy!'

Kate, another sufferer, agreed. 'I never used to take much time to be aware of myself or what I was doing from day to day,' she told me. 'I was probably the perfect example of living an unexamined life! Raising my awareness of my life-style in this very gentle way made me conscious of some behaviour patterns that weren't very helpful – the way I responded to stress, and to being tired, for example. It was keeping the diary of how I *was* living that helped me to see how I could do things better.'

If you keep a diary of what you eat and when you eat, you will be able to track down **food triggers** with comparative ease. If you also record your **feelings** – times of stress and unhappiness, for instance, and incidents which caused tension and anxiety – you will also be able to track down patterns of response in your life: patterns which, like anything else, can be changed if you choose to do so. If you separate everyday things from unusual events, you will be able to see if it's the accumulation of the ordinary or frequent, or if it's adding something out-of-the-ordinary, which triggers an attack.

You will only be able to consider this if you have a full record. Memory is too fragile and subjective a thing to serve you in this search.

The best method and layout to choose is something that's easy for you to fill in, and easy to recover information from. I have three different suggestions to make. The chances are that one will suit you better than the others.

1. A headache and migraine diary

This is definitely better than no record at all – and if it sounds as though I'm damning it with faint praise, that's not really true!

If the idea of keeping a fully fledged diary intimidates you before you've even started, then just recording your headaches and migraines may be a very good place to start. It's certainly useful if you are experiencing other headaches as well as migraine, or if you suspect the pattern of the headaches you are having is changing in some way.

As a minimum, you should record the **days**, and the **times of day** on which your headaches or migraines occur. ('H' = headache and 'M' = migraine.) Say **how long** they last, and **how bad** they were (mild, moderate, or awful). Did you **feel sick** and/or vomit? What **medication** did you take for it – how many pills, and when? Did you try other **treatments** like hot- or cold-packs; sleep; relaxation; and so forth? Women should also include the details of their **menstrual cycle**.

All this will help you to identify the best remedies, and it will also be an excellent record to present to your doctor if you want to ask for medical help, or for a referral to a specialist.

The main disadvantage of keeping a diary only of the headaches themselves is that it is much more difficult to remember details from the day before a migraine attack begins – let alone from the day before that! Sometimes, it is those very details which provide the key to the attack, and so your solution may be delayed if you are alerted only after the attacks begin.

Still, if the answer *does* lie in the immediate situation surrounding the onset of the migraine, your work will

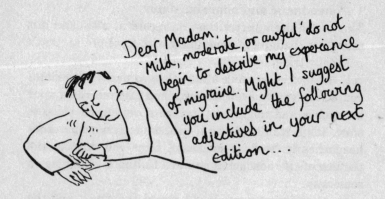

Dear Madam,
'Mild, moderate, or awful' do not begin to describe my experience of migraine. Might I suggest you include the following adjectives in your next edition ...

bear fruit. Or you may begin with a simple headache diary, and discover after some weeks that insufficient evidence is being collected. Then you will have built up a good history of note-taking, and be in an excellent position to extend the range of information with a fuller record.

2. A daily chart

You can get a free sample of an outline chart of this sort from the Migraine Trust in London, and from several drug companies such as Roche Nicholas, the manufacturer of Femigraine. Down one side of the sheet are listed the hours of the day, and along the top of the sheet are specific events which are relevant to tracking down migraine triggers and treatment, such as travel, exercise, food and drink, warning signs, medications, bed-times, and so on. You simply tick off the items which apply each day, and make brief notes about the details. And, of course, you can either use photocopies of the printed suggestions, or you can rule up your own chart.

114

I have two inter-connected criticisms of this sort of record, and although you may have your own solutions for them, I do want just to point them out.

It is quite difficult to use a chart of this kind which has been created by someone else to cover general probabilities instead of your own personal realities. I filled one chart in for three weeks before I gave up, because I couldn't make sense of *my* life in relationship to the headings. I may have been unconsciously creating problems for myself to try to avoid the burden of recording anything at all, but for whatever reason, the chart and I were just not well suited.

'So make up your own chart!' I hear you cry. 'It'll still be easier than starting from a blank page!'

And it may be. But the trouble with that is that *you* will then have decided in advance what categories of information you will record, and so you may completely miss some other factor – something you'd never thought of in connection with your migraine.

However, if this idea appeals to you, it makes sense to try it out. Here are the sorts of headings you should consider including, when you set up your record.

Food/when eaten Don't forget to include snacks; you're trying to identify both the food you consume, and the times at which you do so. Be specific.

Medication/what taken/when taken Include everything you take, no matter what it's for or how benign you believe it to be. And don't forget to include anything you take for migraine.

Drink/when drunk Record everything you drink: mineral water, tea and coffee (many of us forget the ones we

115

automatically consume at work, but you must include those). Note whether or not you have milk, and sweeteners of any kind. Note the sort of wine, the brand of soda, and so forth. That way, you can change brands if you suspect a specific culprit.

Menstrual cycle   Women should keep a record of their menstrual cycle, so they can trace its connections with migraine attacks. Time it from the first day of your period.

Sleep patterns   Sleeping well or badly is an important record to keep. If the amount of time you spend sleeping is important to you, record that in hours, and say how you felt when you woke up. Still tired? Headachy? Fresh and full of bounce? Rate it on a scale if that makes the entry easier – say, 'A' for a full eight hours and feeling full of beans when you wake; and so on.

Good and bad moments   Again, these can be rated in a scale of feelings in as brief a form as you like, but it is very important to keep a record of them in some way. If you have a phone call that fills you with elation or despair, put it down. If you have a shouting-match with your spouse or your boss or your children, say so. If you feel especially competent or happy or successful or contented, then add that. Include long-term problems, too, and how you're coping with them. The shock of a loved one's death; the breakdown of relationships; a deadly job: all such things bring great stress. And so can happy ones, like falling in love!

Notice yourself – and keep a record of what you notice.

Migraine attacks   You will need to record as much

detail as you can about each attack: the stages, how long each part lasts, what it involves, what seemed to help, and when it eased.

With this evidence gathered over several months, you will stand an excellent chance of putting it into context: what happened just before; whether there are links between this migraine and others in the recent past; and whether or not you can – looking back – see what might have triggered it.

3. Keeping a full diary
This is the one I recommend, especially if your trigger factors seem especially mysterious. There are two basic ways to approach it.

BUILD IT INTO AN EXISTING ROUTINE
If you already use a desk diary at work, and there's enough room to add a migraine record to it, use that. You'll be able to incorporate detailing the required information into your usual daily routines, and it won't be hard to do.

'I had never kept any sort of detailed diary before, and I knew I would find it hard,' Kay told me. 'So I used my desk diary, and entered the things I thought I needed to keep track of, every morning as soon as I got to work. I had a marker in the diary with a code on it, so that I didn't have to use up too much diary space with the entries, and so that anyone referring to my diary at the office didn't instantly have access to my private problem! I kept the entries very simple. The food was important; the times of eating were important; and I also put down a record of the sort of extremes of feelings I'd had that day: highs and lows; any moments of real stress or tension that had made me feel very anxious, or sick. I kept that up for four months without a break, and by then I had had five migraine attacks, and I could identify several patterns which I could do something about.'

DIVIDE THE RECORD INTO TWO PARTS

This suggestion comes from the Leicester Migraine Self-Help Group, and it's both simple and very easy to do.

'Keep a brief record of your day, each day,' advised Lynda. 'Don't worry about doing it at the same time each day – just do it when you can find a free minute. The important thing is to divide the record into two parts: the regular, ordinary things, and the unusual things. You might do this on facing pages in a notebook, or you might use one of those large page-a-day diaries, and use the top and the bottom half of each page for the two parts.

'So at the top you might say what time you got up and what you ate and when you ate it, and so on. Then, in the second part, you put down the unusual events of the day – a party, or seeing a particular person, or your period starting, or eating out in a restaurant: whatever's out of the ordinary.

'Don't look at the diary for several months – just fill it in and tuck it away each day.

'Then go through it with a highlighter pen in your hand, and mark anything – from either section – that reoccurs. You are probably looking for out-of-the-ordinary things which cluster around the days before a migraine, so concentrate on those. But don't neglect the ordinary as well: sometimes they can have a cumulative effect.'

You do have to keep up the diary day after day – even when you don't feel like recording anything, and you don't think it's any use, either. So it involves making a commitment. And it won't be a good record if you wait until the end of the week, or even just a few days, and then write down what you remember!

CALLING IN THE EXPERTS

Once you have assembled some evidence, you can ask for expert help about it. Your doctor is one of these experts, and even though you'll have already seen your GP for the initial diagnosis, now's the time to ask again: for referral, perhaps, or for specific guidance. There are others to consider as well. Whom you see, and what you ask them, will be partly determined by what you have discovered, or suspect, about your migraines.

The dentist

There are two possible dentally related reasons to consult a dentist about migraine. The first is to have your '**bite**' checked, because some migraine attacks as well as other sorts of head pain can be triggered by a defect in the way your top teeth meet your bottom teeth when you bite on food. If there is a misalignment of some kind which is causing an asymmetrical bite, it is usually simple to correct. It is also possible that **tooth decay**, or **impacted wisdom teeth**, may be the cause of your problems, and a thorough dental check-up, which will probably include an X-ray, should be able to identify any of these causes.

There is also some recent evidence to suggest that at least some migraines are caused by sufferers unconsciously 'grinding' their teeth in their sleep. If you suspect you suffer from this (and your family or spouse may be able to confirm it), then it's definitely worth following up. **Teeth-clenching** and **grinding** can cause muscular spasms in the jaw, and it is the spasms which may trigger morning migraine. Your dentist may be able to fit a simple **splint** over your back teeth, which when worn at night prevents the grinding movements.

I have heard two reports of people using such a splint. One finds the mouth plate very difficult to tolerate and isn't yet sure of any benefit; but the other believes it has completely cured her migraines.

Neck and spine manipulators

If you associate your migraine attacks with pain in your neck or the upper part of your back, then your **muscular pain** may be related to even a minor mis-alignment in your spine, which may well respond to treatment from a physiotherapist, an osteopath, or a chiropractor. And a disturbance of the bones in your neck can cause pain in your eyes and forehead – it's called referred pain.

The muscular pain, of course, may be caused by tension – and will probably be alleviated by **relaxation exercises**, whatever the cause – but it makes good sense to consult a specialist, especially if the pain or stiffness persists beyond the migraine attack's time-span. Again, of course, you will have to start with your own doctor if you want a referral. Before you turn to Chapter Seven, and considering alternative treatments, do discuss physiotherapy with your doctor – for this should be available through the NHS. A good physiotherapist can often correct specific muscle, tendon and ligament problems. They can also help with exercises to alleviate back and neck pain.

Your own doctor

You are lucky if your GP responds in a positive and informed way to migraine. The experience of many migraine sufferers is a dismal one when it comes to consultation – so dismal, in fact, that many have not talked to anyone in the medical profession about their condition for years.

'I had thirty years of failure with doctors,' said one migraineur. 'It seems to me that if a doctor doesn't manage to cure whatever you have, they feel ineffectual and resentful.'

If *your* doctor responds in a helpful and positive way to your condition, then treasure them! If they do not, you will need to encourage them to do better. Present yourself in the right way, and you will stand a much better chance of attracting respect and attention.

In Britain, many doctors' surgeries organise the appointments system so that only seven and a half minutes are allowed for each appointment. That will not be enough time to discuss your migraines, so ask the receptionist if you can book a double appointment slot, or take the last appointment of the morning or afternoon – whichever solution they prefer.

It will also help if you have a clear idea of your symptoms, and what you want to achieve, before you visit the doctor. Your diary record will make an excellent start to this programme.

Even if you have not yet gathered enough evidence from a diary, you should be able to answer most of the following questions. Do make notes in advance and take these with you to the surgery, or you will run the risk of forgetting some of the details.

121

QUESTIONS YOUR DOCTOR MAY ASK YOU

★ **When did the migraines begin?** In childhood – or last year? Did they start when your periods began? Or when you moved house or job? This sort of information will help your doctor to build up a clear picture of your problem, and the possible lines of treatment.

★ **How often do the attacks occur, and how long do they last?** Does this vary from time to time? Have they got worse, or better, over time? Has this affected your decision to consult the doctor, or is there another factor involved?

★ **Where does the pain begin?** Does it move around, or change, during the attack? Does anything (like movement, for example) make it worse or better?

★ **What seems to bring the headaches on? What precedes them?**

★ **Do any other symptoms accompany the headaches?** Do you have nausea or other gastric disturbances with the headache? Do you get flashing lights, or a loss of vision, or increased sensitivity to light or sound or smells, with the headache?

★ **What makes the headaches better?** Is it just time, or does a particular treatment help? Does heat, or cold, or anything else, help? Have your tried relaxation?

★ **What effect does this have on your life?** If you are losing days from work, or if your family is responding badly to your condition, now is the time to say so. Migraine is not life-threatening, but it can play havoc with the quality of your life, and that's very important.

WHAT DO YOU EXPECT THE DOCTOR TO DO?

It's a good idea to ask yourself in advance what you expect from the consultation. If you want a referral to a specialist service such as a migraine clinic, or a physiotherapist, you will need to be clear about why you want that, and be prepared to defend your request. If you want to find out what treatments are available, you should consider whether you are looking for something that will alleviate the painful and unpleasant effects of an attack, or whether you want something to prevent the attacks from happening in the first place.

Perhaps you are looking for a more effective drug, or one with fewer (or less distressing) side-effects. There is a detailed list of the various **drug treatments** available for migraine in Chapter Six, with a note of their main effects – and possible side-effects – so that you can check your own treatments against an understanding of what is presently available to you. But drug choices are determined by many different factors, and your doctor is qualified to weigh these up, and make decisions in the light of all of them, in discussion with you.

DRUG TREATMENTS

You should never take any medicine without understanding what its effects are supposed to be; what its side-effects might be; and without checking the contra-indications (the specific reasons why the drug might not be suitable for you) with a doctor.

There are a number of medical conditions which make certain drugs unsuitable for use: diabetes, certain heart conditions, asthma and chronic bronchitis are some obvious examples. Your doctor will have a record of your medical condition, of course, and so will be able to prescribe in the light of that information. But perhaps you may have some other information which is relevant. Family history? A suspicion that a particular medication is causing an unpleasant side-effect? Make a note to tell your doctor.

You may also seek your doctor's support in a particular form of self-help treatment, such as a **food exclusion diet** (see pages 63 to 70 and 179). The ideal situation is to obtain your GP's help and support in your efforts to control, to minimise or to defeat your condition. With that support, your chances of success are good. Without it, your task is more difficult – but it is by no means impossible. If you can work out how to get your doctor on your side – interested in your problem and fighting alongside you in your efforts – your struggle will be an easier one.

There are also some basic ways to help yourself, without necessarily calling in the professionals. Trying some acupressure yourself, at home, is one to consider.

PUTTING ON THE PRESSURE

I found out about pressure points and relief from migraine pain quite by chance, during a bad migraine attack a year or so ago. As the pain and nausea was reaching its height, I noticed an especially tender and aching point near my left shoulder blade.

When that point was pressed, the pain was at first much worse – but it was also in some way a relief, much like pressing on an aching tooth, or on a bruise. And it certainly helped: the headache pain eased, my nose cleared, and I was able to sleep off the remaining effects of the migraine attack successfully. Since then, I have found excellent results from regular pressure-point massage for avoiding migraine, and any attack which does slip through is milder and more responsive to relaxation techniques. I just wish I could reach that critical spot myself!

You can, of course, visit a masseur or an acupuncturist to have pressure-point treatments of various kinds, but you can also do it yourself, on four pairs of pressure points which give you access to headache-related nerves. These are near your eyes; on your neck; near your thumbs; and lastly, on your wrists.

With a bit of practice, applying pressure to the right spots can bring effective relief from pain, and it can stop a migraine attack in its tracks before the pain has had a chance to get established. The advantages of self-applied acupressure are that it is perfectly safe, genuinely effective, and relatively simple and straight-forward to do.

It has two potential disadvantages: it can be quite tricky to find exactly the right spots (but you do know when you have found one); and the points are always rather sensitive, even when you *don't* have a headache. When you have head pain, pressing hard on the pressure points will be very uncomfortable – and hard pressure is the best way to get results. A few seconds of pain is much preferable to hours or days of headache – but you have to believe that to press hard!

Because there is a remote suspicion of danger in apply-ing pressure to some nerves during **pregnancy**, you should not attempt *any* of this if you are pregnant. But

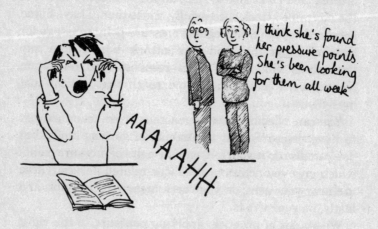

since the chances are that if you are pregnant, your migraines will have disappeared, that news is not as depressing as it might seem!

Applying the right pressure

In order for the technique to work well, you have to apply a hard, constant pressure to a small area. You should make the pressure point *hurt*: for a short time, admittedly, but it is still pain.

Counting to ten, or maybe to fifteen (depending on how fast you're counting), is about right. You can try taking a series of slow, calm breaths – five in, five out. You can press hard for a count of five, ease off the pressure for the count of five, and then press again – or you can use a steady, firm pressure (and get it over with). Some experts suggest using your thumbnail, but don't do that if your nail is long or sharp, because you must not press so hard that you damage your skin. Be firm, not timid, but don't overdo it.

Press the points in pairs
Even if it seems as though only one of a pair of pressure points is tender, you should press on both points in a pair. You can do the ones on your head and neck simultaneously, but of course you will need to press the ones on your hands one after the other.

You need to treat both points because you are pressing the two branches of the same part of the nerve, and you will get much better and more reliable results from dealing with the whole, rather than with just one half of it.

You'll know when you've found it
Locating the precise point can be rather tricky: some people can do it almost immediately; others take much longer. You need to be patient, and you need to move your thumb or your finger – whichever you are using – very slowly and methodically over a tiny area, pressing carefully as you go.

You will certainly know when you find the right point! If you press correctly, then you are pressing directly on a place where the nerve is accessible to pressure, and close to the surface of the skin. If you are even just a centimetre off-target, you won't be able to get enough pressure on the nerve to make much difference to your headache.

The right spot feels extremely sensitive when you press on it, even when you don't have a headache. It may feel a bit odd – a sort of combination of pain and numbness or tingling – and the sensation feels as though it is travelling away from the spot.

Getting to the points
Practise this when you do *not* have a migraine!

Hands first Spread one hand out (your left hand if you
are right-handed, and vice versa) palm down, on a flat
surface, and look at it. There is a sort of triangle of flesh
between your thumb and your index finger. Spread your
hand a little more, so that the 'web' is stretched as flat as
possible.

The point you are searching for is within that web,
against the bone of your index finger, near the middle of it
on the thumb side. Push your other thumb in against that
index-finger bone. Move the nail or the tip of your thumb
– whichever you are using – back and forth, moving just a
little at a time. You will find a tender, sensitive spot,
which will give you a tiny jolt of pain, quite different from
any pressure a little further away. You are now pressing
on the nerve. Well done.

Then repeat the exercise on the other hand. Make sure
you get the same sort of feeling on both hands.

Go on to your wrists Spread out your hand again, and
look further down, towards your wrist, on the thumb side.
You may be able to see a small bump of bone at the top of
your forearm, where your wrist joins your hand.

If you can't see it, you will certainly be able to feel it
with the thumb of your other hand. Run your thumb up
that last part of your arm, and feel the bump at the end
of the bone. (The radius, which is the bone on the thumb
side of your arm, ends with the bump you are looking
for.)

Above the bump, still on the thumb side, there is a
small dip. In the dip is the point you are looking for.

Push down into the dip with the tip of your thumb, or with your thumbnail. There should be a real sensitivity, a feeling of a travelling pain which goes up into your hand, or down into your arm.

Some people find this a hard point to discover. Keep trying, moving your thumb around and along the area. Or leave this one and come back to it, once you have found other points and know exactly how to identify the sensation you seek.

Try the back of your neck Put one hand on the back of your neck, and feel with the tip of one finger for the place where your skull joins your neck. You will find that there is a bony ridge just behind each ear. If you run the tips of your fingers along the base of your skull, in from the ridge, and towards the middle of your neck, your fingertips will reach a muscular 'dip' in the middle of the back of your neck.

Now, retrace your fingertip journey. Halfway between the ridge behind your ear, and the groove in the middle of the back of your neck, there is another smaller groove between two muscles. You might find it easier to find this spot if you push your chin forward on to your chest, and so tighten the muscles at the back of your neck.

Once you have found the smaller groove, run the tip of your thumb, or your index finger, up this groove to the base of your skull. Press hard up against the bone, and into the groove. When you feel the intense sensitivity or tingling pain, you will know you have found the right spot.

The eyes have it A mirror is very helpful for finding this last pair of pressure points.

Run your index finger gently and carefully along the edge of the bone above your eye socket, until you reach the outer corner. Now look in the mirror, and run your finger slowly up the ridge of bone, towards the end of your eyebrow. When you have got about halfway, roll your finger back towards your ear, and you will find that it travels over the surface of the ridge of bone. Here you will feel a small depression in the bone; press hard to find the exact spot of the nerve.

If you have brought your finger all the way back into the hollow in your temple, you have gone too far. Take your finger back to the edge of your eye socket, and try again.

When to use auto-acupressure

★   Do it when the headache first starts. Don't wait until the pain gets worse – it will be harder to treat by any method if you wait.

★   Do it anywhere. This is one of the great advantages of acupressure; you really can do it anywhere, without people necessarily noticing, and without your drawing attention to yourself and your problem. The hand and wrist points, in particular, are useful in such situations. The eye and neck ones can easily be treated while you're sitting at your desk at work.

★   Repeating the pressure is perfectly safe. If you start with them in the order listed above, and find any pair more successful or helpful, then any repeat treatments can concentrate on those points.

LIE BACK AND RELAX

If you are convinced that there is a physical cause for your migraines, you will probably want to dismiss the idea that **relaxation techniques** could help you. Or maybe you lead such a difficult and stressful life that you don't see how to find time for relaxation exercises, let alone the idea of **self-hypnosis**.

The truth is that most people don't realise just how stressed they are, until they start to relax. Most of us don't become conscious of how tense certain muscles are until we have a go at relaxing them.

Relaxation techniques won't just help your migraine when the attacks begin; they will also help you to cope with the whole spectrum of life's trials and triumphs in a more balanced and easy way. You can always find time to fit in what you want to do, so the trick, here, is first to decide that you want to try it out.

If the very idea of relaxing sets your teeth on edge with anxiety, you might need to start yourself off with some sort of relaxation aid. **Massage sandals** (the sort that have little bumps on the inner sole) might help; so might the **rollers** which you rub your feet across to ease tension (the Body Shop has them). *Stress and Relaxation* by Jane Madders, published by Macdonald, is a very good basic book, especially helpful for migraineurs. And there are lots of different **relaxation tapes** which you could try – your local library's audio department may even have some you could borrow. You can also buy excellent relaxation and **pain control tapes** which you can use when a migraine has struck, as well as for general relaxation (see pages 144 to 145). These can often do much to lessen an attack's severity.

131

'When I wake up with that unmistakable pain behind my right eye,' said Margaret, 'I just switch on the tape-player in my bedside radio – the tape is permanently inside it! If the pain feels very advanced, I also take two aspirin. The tape is so soothing that I drift into a semi-conscious state for a while – not sleep, but close to it. After half an hour or so, the head pain has retreated, and as long as I'm careful, I can cope again.'

Do-it-yourself starting points
Start off by shutting your eyes for a moment, and attending to your body. You may think you're reasonably relaxed – but is that really true?

1. Recognise the physical signs of stress

Head and neck   Is your jaw clenched, even though you are just sitting, doing nothing much at all? Are your teeth firmly clenched? Are your lips tightly closed, rather than just closed? Is your tongue pressed tight against the roof of your mouth? Are your eyes either pressed wide open, or screwed up?

Where is your head – pushed forward? Bent down? Are your neck muscles tight or stiff from keeping it there?

Arms and hands   Are your shoulders hunched forward, or up towards your ears? Are your upper arms clenched in against your chest? Are your hands clenched?

Legs and feet   Do you wind one leg around the other? Do you sit with your toes clenched?

Body pattern   Do you sit with your whole body tensed

forward and rigid? Do you get a lot of back pain?

Breathing Do you notice the inward breaths you take, more than any other? Do you sigh a lot? Do your breathing patterns tend to be irregular, rather than steady?

2. Take control of your own stress patterns

If you recognise yourself in any (or all) of those examples, it is very likely that stress patterns are influencing the frequency or the severity of your migraines. You can begin to change that right now, by learning a new way for your body to behave. If you can achieve a relaxed physical state, your mental state will improve as well. Migraineurs, in particular, should concentrate on relaxation exercises that ease the stress in face, neck and shoulders, but the whole of your body can benefit from attention.

3. Start with your attitude

You could begin by looking at the three most common problems of attitude found amongst those who need to relax. Do you recognise your own problems here? If you do, it's more than time you began to find ways to relieve your anxieties and tensions.

★ **Take it easy** In the eye of eternity, it really doesn't matter if you have forgotten to do something, or done something badly. Take things more slowly, and learn to adopt a long view of things.

★ **Value yourself** You can handle problems as well as anyone else – if you let yourself. Everyone has problems; everyone makes mistakes.

★ **Accept yourself, faults and all** Find a way to talk about your worries, and to admit the things that make you worried or upset.

'I never thought I'd say it,' admitted Paul after reluctantly attending relaxation classes at the local health centre, 'but I feel *much* better equipped to cope with the pressures of life. I was so tangled up in work problems I thought I'd explode. I'd got so close to the problems, I had no way to let them go. But the relaxation exercises helped me to see things differently. I don't want to tempt fate, but I've only had one migraine attack since I did the course, and that was nothing like the old ones I used to get. Maybe I'm cured . . .'

4. Physical relaxation techniques

Breathing Practise breathing in and out as evenly as possible. Take a slow breath in – say, for the count of six; hold it for the count of two, and then breathe out slowly, say for the count of eight, trying to get rid of all of the breath you took in. Count two, and then do it again.

After ten of these slow in-and-out breaths, start to attend to *where* you are breathing. Concentrate on making the breathing centre on your stomach, rather than your chest. Push your stomach *out* as you breathe *in*; pull your stomach *in* as you breathe *out*.

Identify the tension Once your breathing is easy and relaxed, you can start to tackle the tension in other parts of your body. Pick just one example which you identified from the list above of typical tensions. Maybe your shoulders will be a good place to begin.

Exaggerate the tension First, tense your shoulders right up; make it as extreme an example of a tense shoulder position as you can manage. Concentrate on it; really feel that tension as you hunch your shoulders up towards your ears.

Reverse the direction of the tension Now *reverse* the action. Don't just relax your shoulders back to where you think the muscles will be at rest; reverse the tension in the other direction. So tell yourself to pull your shoulders down towards the ground – and do it. Stretch as hard as you can in that tense position.

Relax the tension And then you can relax. Tell the muscles to stop pulling, and roll your shoulders around a little until you find the position of maximum comfort and ease.

Feel the relaxation Consciously feel how your shoulders are, when they are at ease, with the muscles ready to act, but at rest. Stay with that feeling for a few seconds, before you move on to the next exercise.

HOW TO USE RELAXATION TECHNIQUES

Often it isn't until you stop doing something that you realise you were doing it at all – and that's certainly the case with muscle tension of this sort. In order to combat it successfully you will have to allow yourself some time on a regular basis to practise relaxation: first, by easing the tension in the ways described above, and secondly, to promote some positive counter-tension exercises for your mind and your body.

Room for manoeuvre

You allow yourself time for meals, for washing and dressing, and for sleep, so you can certainly allow yourself some relaxation time if you choose to do so. The ideal is probably about thirty minutes, but ten minutes is a great deal better than no time at all. You can make ten minutes a day, easily.

Meditation can certainly help. It's an excellent form of relaxation for migraineurs, especially those with anxious and active minds! If you need help to slow down your thoughts and worries, this is a good way to do it.

'Meditation taught me how to create a mental space for myself where I was in control,' said Robert. 'I could make a sort of gap stretch out in my mind, between myself and what was happening to me at work. Thinking like that helped me see that I *could* control things, and that helped my attitude towards my migraines. Which helped me to tackle them. It was like a chain of command, with me in charge of myself.'

To start with you will need some space that won't be invaded by other people, that's relatively warm, and in which you can either lie on the floor or lean back in a chair. If you can also find a space that's fairly quiet, it will help – but it's unrealistic to look for somewhere that's sound-proofed from the world. In any case, you will soon learn to cut out the distraction-effect of background noise. And you will eventually be able to do this almost anywhere.

One person I know manages self-hypnosis on the London Underground, speeding along between appointments; another happily practises meditation on the exercise bike at the gym! That's the ideal – a technique which allows you to cope well within the real, noisy, smelly world. I'm not that proficient (yet), so I still need to shut myself away.

1. In the beginning

Lie down on the floor, or lean back in your chair. Make yourself as comfortable as you can. Put a pillow behind your head, or squash up a small pillow so it supports just your neck. Have your legs straight (don't cross them), and have your arms on the armrests of the chair, or rest them on your thighs, or put your arms by your sides with your hands lightly on your stomach.

Start with your feet, and travel up your body to your head. At each part of you, put into practice the 'tense it/reverse it/relax it' technique explained above.

So, for example, with your feet. Start by tensing your toes; but start gently, or you may go straight to a cramp, and have to use up the rest of your relaxation time hopping around releasing the jammed muscles! Then reverse the tension; flex your toes back up. Hold each position long enough to feel and experience it; be aware of what your muscles are doing, and how they feel when they are like that.

Then, deliberately, release the tension. Relax your feet. Feel the relaxation.

Now do the same with your legs. Scrunch the muscles up, reverse the tension back the other way, then release it completely.

Follow this pattern up through your body, making sure that in the process you involve all the muscles you know about.

When you have finished, close your eyes, and lie (or

sit) as peacefully as you can, for a few minutes. Don't screw up your eyes; *relax* them shut. Do five in, five out breaths again, as you did to start with. By now, they will come much more easily, regularly, and enjoyably.

2. CONCENTRATE ON PROBLEM AREAS

Because **muscle tension** in your face, neck, and shoulders is known to be a possible migraine trigger, it makes excellent sense to develop some exercises specifically for those areas. Here are some to try. They're quick and simple, and you can do them in between tasks, while you're waiting for someone to answer the telephone, at the traffic lights . . .

Shoulders Bring your shoulders right up to your ears – really scrunch them up tense and tight. Hold them there for the count of five – and then let them go. Repeat twice. Then rotate them: five times forwards, and five times back.

Do the same exercise again, but this time moving each shoulder singly instead of together.

Back and shoulders Bring your forearms together in front of your chest, so that they are parallel from wrists to elbows. Then, leading with your wrists, make circles in the air. Imagine a pen tied to each wrist if that helps: the lines which the two pens draw in front of you should just touch in front of your chest, each time you make the circles. Repeat this twice, and then reverse the direction of the circles.

Clasp your hands on your elbows out in front of your chest, so that your arms form three sides of a square, and your body forms the fourth side. Raise your arms up to the level of your nose; hold them there for the count of five, and then bring them back to chest height. Repeat.

Neck   Stand as relaxed as you can, and bring your chin right down to your chest. Then, gently and slowly, bring your chin around in a 'circle' so that your neck rotates. Don't move your body; just try to move your neck. You will probably find that there are bits of the 'circle' which feel especially stiff, but don't force it. Just keep the movement as slow and easy as you can, and skip the parts you can't manage (you'll get better). Repeat the 'circle' in the opposite direction.

Start with your head in its normal position, and then bring your head right down in the same way as before, with your chin dropped forward on your chest. Then lift your head right back, so that your chin is stretched up towards the ceiling. Bring your head upright again, and then drop it slowly down towards your right shoulder. Move only your head; don't bring your shoulder up to help the process along, and don't try to force your head further than feels comfortable. Take it slowly and easily; it's not a competition.

Arms and shoulders   Shake your arms out and away from your body. Try shaking each part of your arm – your hands, and then your hands and forearms, and then your hands and the whole of your arms – keeping the muscles as limp and free as you can.

SELF-HYPNOSIS

There is a section on hypnosis in Chapter Seven, and it is a form of self help that I thoroughly recommend. One advantage is that the technique of self-hypnosis is quite easy to master, and once you have done that, it is a self-help technique which you can put into practice almost anywhere and any time to reduce the effects of stress in your life.

Self-hypnosis involves learning a physical relaxation technique such as the one above, where you begin with your feet and move up through your body, relaxing every muscle. When that's achieved, you can learn **visualisation techniques** to induce a deep mental relaxation as well. Some people learn to imagine themselves descending a staircase, step by step: at the bottom of the staircase they can find their own chosen private world – the place they would most like to be. I take particular enjoyment in the last moment at the top of the staircase, where I have been taught to take any problem that's bothering me – a person, a task or a situation – and drop it firmly into a basket before starting down the stairs!

The best results will come from learning self-hypnosis from a reputable and properly qualified hypnotist whom you respect and trust. Look at the recommendations in Chapter Seven.

FEVERFEW

You may have heard, or read, of the excellent results many migraine sufferers have found through taking a herb called feverfew. Clinical trials have repeated the success found by many individuals, and the herb has now been given a scientific 'seal of approval'. It should not, however, be taken by pregnant women.

How does it work?

Feverfew's active ingredients act on the platelets in your blood, and inhibit the release of serotonin from the platelets. It is serotonin which may trigger migraine attacks through its effects on blood flow (see pages 36 to 37).

Grow it yourself

Feverfew is a common perennial garden plant. You may already have it in your garden, or have seen it growing. There are, however, different varieties of feverfew, and it is only one sort, the wild variety of the plant, called *Tanacetum parthenium*, which is helpful. This variety has light green, rather feathery leaves, and daisy-like flowers which are yellow in the centre with white outer petals.

If you want to try to grow fresh feverfew to take for migraine, do make quite sure you are buying – or being given – the right plant. If you are in any doubt, buy your seeds or your plants from an established and reputable herb farm or seed merchant. The real feverfew is a safe herb, which is taken on a daily basis by thousands of people, so that's the one you need. Don't run the risk of taking the wrong plant, which may have no effect at all – or, worse still, some other unpleasant effects.

Feverfew isn't a particularly fussy plant, and it will grow in any soil, although it prefers a semi-shaded position. You need to grow more than one plant to ensure a ready supply of fresh leaves. Grow three or four plants together, and pinch out the flower buds from all but one of the plants (if you allow one to flower, you can save seeds for new, replacement plants in the future).

Using feverfew leaves

Feverfew is taken as a preventative for migraine, and the usual dose needed is two or three small leaves every day. Some people find that if they take the leaves constantly for three months, they have a further migraine-free period after they stop, without having to take more feverfew. Other people find that the herb lessens the severity of the headaches, or that it cuts down on nausea and vomiting.

Feverfew smells pleasantly aromatic, but the leaves do taste bitter – and some people find that they get slight mouth ulcers, or an itchy effect in their mouths. If that happens, you should stop taking it; the symptoms will disappear in a day.

To guard against the side-effects, and to mask the bitterness of the taste, you can try eating the leaves inside a sandwich. One woman I read about wrapped the feverfew inside lettuce leaves as well.

Dried feverfew seems to work just as well as fresh, but don't try an infusion of the dried leaves as a drink, because it's too hard to control the dose.

Feverfew in tablet form

You can buy feverfew tablets in most health food shops, and in many chemist shops. Herbal Laboratories' Herbal Feverfew 125 (one 125mg tablet a day) has been recommended, and so have Heath and Heather's tablets (two 25mg tablets a day).

Many people find that taking tablets is much easier than cultivating and maintaining plants in their gardens.

The dose is already calculated and measured out for you, and the risk of mouth ulcers is much reduced (as is the unpleasant taste).

VITAMINS AND OTHER SUPPLEMENTS

We are often told that vitamin supplements are an unnecessary and expensive addition to our diets, and that may well be true. On the other hand, migraine sufferers who elaborately try to avoid various foods, and who also vomit or have other digestive upsets, may be especially vulnerable to the loss or lack of certain foods. It's certainly worth considering.

Vitamin B6 (pyridoxine) is often prescribed for premenstrual tension, and it is also recommended for women whose migraines are menstrual, or menstrually related. You do need to take the correct dose with this vitamin, for overdosing can have dangerous effects, and the side-effects of excess doses of vitamin B6 include, ironically enough, headaches and nausea . . .

So be sure never to exceed 500mg a day, and remember that vitamin B6 is best if balanced with other B vitamins and with magnesium (so consider a B-complex supplement if you want to try this treatment). Look for a yeast-free version of vitamin B pills if you suspect that yeast may be a migraine trigger for you. Natural sources of vitamin B6 include **brewer's yeast, wheat bran** and **wheat germ, liver** and **kidney, cabbage**, and **cantaloupe melon**.

Niacin, another member of the B-complex family, is also known as vitamin B3, and amongst its functions is the synthesis of insulin. Some people find taking supplements of this can reduce the severity of migraines. Natural sources include **liver, wholewheat products, fish, eggs, dates, figs** and **prunes**. If you are already taking a B-complex pill or a multi-vitamin, check the label – niacin is probably included.

Oil of Evening Primrose has its strong adherents and supporters amongst migraine sufferers, and especially amongst those whose migraines are hormonally triggered. This oil is high in an essential fatty acid known as gamma linolenic acid (GLA for short), which plays an important role in maintaining the levels of prostaglandins – natural chemicals which regulate the effects of female hormones during the menstrual cycle.

A new alternative to Evening Primrose Oil is called **Starflower Oil** – extracted from borage flowers. It contains much more concentrated GLA, and so you need to take fewer capsules to achieve the same results, which should also work out cheaper.

Quick tips to consider

★ Avoid hunger.
★ Exercise regularly, but in moderate ways.
★ Avoid positions which cause muscle strain.
★ Avoid habitual contraction of face and jaw muscles.
★ Learn some simple relaxation techniques and put those into practice when you feel tense or anxious.
★ Adjust your life to deal with stress levels.

USEFUL ADDRESSES
The Pain Relief Foundation, Rice Lane, Liverpool, has a tape available called *Coping with Headaches and Migraine*, which currently costs £7.55 including postage

and packing. Send a stamped addressed envelope with any enquiries.

Health and Well-being is a self-hypnosis relaxation tape designed in conjunction with the Leicester Migraine Self-Help Group, by Peter Delves. Send £4.95 plus 70p postage and packing to Peter Delves, 40 Houlditch Road, Clarendon Park, Leicester LE2 3FE.

Managing Migraine is a free service run by Glaxo Laboratories Ltd, and includes a relaxation tape. Write to Managing Migraine, Freepost, PO Box 21, Godalming, Surrey GU17 2BR, or telephone (0272) 767644.

CHAPTER 6

Conventional
Drug Treatments

Conventional drugs tend to get a bad press these days, and we often worry about the effects of 'pill-popping' on our minds and bodies. 'I feel like a pain-killer junkie,' one migraineur told me, whilst another longed to find a way of weaning herself off the drugs she used.

Some migraine sufferers also feel cynical about the readiness of GPs to prescribe them away from the surgery. 'As soon as I walk into my doctor's room, I see him pull the prescription pad towards him across the desk,' said Margaret. 'That's his greeting to me! I might be going to ask him for a new prescription, but I'd be happier if he waited to find out – or if I thought he would seriously consider something else instead.'

We are right to be concerned about possible side-effects, for all drugs, over-the-counter or on prescription, can have unpleasant side-effects for some people. And all drugs, however readily available, should be treated with respect and caution. Their effects and their possible side-effects should be known to you before you start. You should thoroughly understand why you have been prescribed them, and how to use them.

But it would be wrong to dismiss modern drugs out of hand because of their potential danger. The relief which is available for migraine sufferers through modern drug research is both astounding and varied. As with so much else in migraine self help, the key to success is in your own hands – and once again you will need to marshal your resources to cope. Don't be intimidated, and don't be a guinea-pig unless you *choose* to be one!

Write it down!

If you want to try out a particular migraine drug treatment, but you are worried about the possible side-effects, *say so to your doctor*. Look back at Chapter Five's section on consulting the experts, and make sure you're well prepared, but do remember that not all migraine treatments are suitable for everyone. Your doctor can tell you which ones are safe for you to try.

Take a pad and pencil with you to the surgery, and *write down* the possible side-effects of what you are prescribed; that way you won't have to try to remember them, weeks later, if you suspect a problem is developing. Ask your doctor what the dangers might be. Ask if there is any food, or any other medication, that you should avoid while you are trying the migraine treatment. *Write down the answers*. Ask about the alternatives. Make sure you understand what you are being told.

'The doctor can't help'

And there is another potential difficulty for migraineurs: many become all too accustomed to their condition. 'The doctor can't do anything about it' is a common statement, even from people who haven't

147

visited their GP in years, or perhaps have never asked about new migraine treatments. So pain and discomfort are endured, in ignorance of possible help.

Most people who manage to affect their migraines in a positive way do so at least partly through the use of drugs. This may mean no more than finding the right pain-killer (often a simple over-the-counter preparation), and taking that when pain begins, or it may mean using a preventative drug on a daily basis, to stop the migraine from occurring.

Talk it through

This chapter outlines the main drug options which are available. But it cannot recommend one preparation over

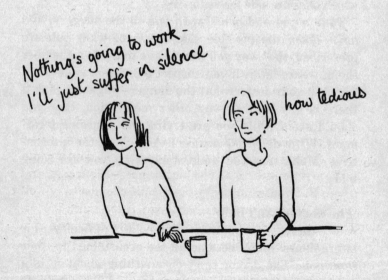

another, because migraine has such a wide range of different manifestations in different people. Only you will be able to decide what works best for you – through trial and error, through thought and discussion, and through your own preferences and choices.

Don't use this information as a substitute for proper detailed discussion with your doctor; rather, use it to help you have that discussion, and to understand more clearly what the options you are offered will mean.

A drug by any other name?

Some people are confused by the different names for drugs, and wonder why the same preparation can be referred to in two or three different ways. In fact, this is a process with which we are already familiar in everyday life.

Every drug has three names: a chemical name, a generic name, and a trade or brand name. Food names, for example, can work in exactly the same way: whole-wheat flour could be referred to by listing the chemical constituents of flour; by naming it generically as flour; or by naming the brand of wholewheat flour which is prepared for commercial sale.

So it is with medical drugs. You will probably never come across the **chemical name** of a drug – it would be a long string of words, letters and numbers, and it could include reference to 'carrier' substances, colourings, and so on. But you, your doctor, and your chemist may well use the **generic name** of a drug when you talk about it. This is the official medical name for the drug, and it is the term used for the basic active substance which it contains.

Next come the **brand names** which drug manufacturers

give their preparations. These names often reflect some of the qualities of the drugs they are selling. Migraine drugs, of course, often include some reference to migraine in their brand names: Imigran, Migraleve, Migravess, and Sanomigran, for example. Cafergot contains both caffeine and ergotamine; Paramax contains both paracetamol and Maxolon – in itself a brand name for an anti-nausea drug with a generic name of metoclopromide.

If a drug is manufactured by more than one company, the generic drug will have several different brand names. And a basic substance like aspirin is often manufactured in combination with other drugs, which means there will be yet more brand names.

With some drugs, it is worth considering what the cheapest form will be. If all you want to use is ibuprofen, for example – an over-the-counter analgesic – then it is sensible to ask the chemist for its cheapest form. But certain combinations of drugs appear only in certain brand-name forms – and, of course, some generic drugs are only produced by one drug company, in one form.

SOME USEFUL TIPS ABOUT TAKING DRUGS

1. Always start with the **stated dose**. Some people tend to begin with less than the recommended dose of a prescribed drug; some people tend to take more than the recommended dose, especially with an over-the-counter analgesic.

Neither of those strategies will produce the best results. If you want to take a very small dose of a prescribed drug, it's best to discuss that possibility with your doctor, rather than just to lower the prescribed amount yourself. Your doctor will know what the lowest *effective* dose of a drug is likely to be. If you take the number of pills that have been prescribed and make a note of the effects, you can then discuss altering the dose with your doctor.

And taking more than the recommended dose of any drug is potentially dangerous. Even over-the-counter pills can have very dangerous effects in overdose.

2.   If you take drugs to deal with the migraine once it begins, **don't wait** until the symptoms get worse. If you get warning signs, take the medication then; if you only know that you have a migraine when the headache begins, don't wait for it to get worse.

Over-the-counter preparations, in particular, work best when they are taken early. They can only deal with pain

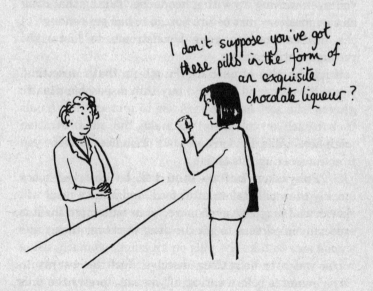

I don't suppose you've got these pills in the form of an exquisite chocolate liqueur?

up to a certain level, and if you leave it until the pain gets worse, the drug may not work at all.

3. If you find **swallowing** pills difficult, ask if there is a smooth capsule, a suppository, a syrup, a nasal spray, a rub-on gel, or an effervescent form of the same drug. Always swallow pills with a big glass of water, so that they can go down quickly and painlessly.

4. Don't automatically dismiss the possibility of taking drugs in a **suppository** form. The British are very coy about using 'botty pills', but in the rest of Europe, drugs are often administered in that way, and it's a positive benefit to migraineurs who are nauseous, or whose stomachs have already 'closed down'. It's also recommended for its fast action in migraine prevention, when taking an anti-migraine drug at night can stop you even waking up with a headache. Taking that drug as a suppository just before you go to bed gets enough of the medication into your bloodstream to last right through until morning.

If it's the idea of pushing the pill up that's upsetting, you can easily (and cheaply) buy thin disposable **plastic gloves** (the sort hairdressers use to protect their hands from bleach or colouring) to make the administration more acceptable. So don't let your prejudices prevent you from considering this option.

5. Pills taken **before food** will be absorbed more quickly than pills taken after food, and a fatty meal will slow down the effects even more. Since with migraine it is especially important to get the drug working quickly, it's a good idea to take the pills on an empty stomach, using warm water to help them dissolve. Wait for twenty to thirty minutes before eating, if you can, to give the pills time to work.

THE MAIN DRUG GROUPS

The main sorts of drugs which are available for migraine treatment are:

★ Ordinary pain-killers (analgesics)
★ Anti-sickness drugs
★ Tranquillisers, and sedatives
★ Anti-depressants
★ Ergotamine
★ Serotonin-antagonists and agonists
★ Beta-blockers
★ Calcium-channel blockers

1. Pain-killers (analgesics)

Aspirin, paracetamol, ibuprofen, and codeine are the most commonly used analgesics, and they are all available in various forms as over-the-counter pills, capsules, and effervescent tablets. It isn't a good idea to mix these drugs together; stick to trying one at a time, until you find the one that works well for you.

Aspirin can be a very effective migraine control, and taking half a soluble aspirin a day can help prevent attacks. On the other hand, it is also a gastric irritant, so it is not recommended for people with stomach ulcers, for asthmatics and other people with a history of allergic reactions, for children under twelve, nor for pregnant women. If you do choose aspirin, try a soluble form, and don't exceed the recommended daily maximum of 4g.

Paracetamol is less of an irritant than aspirin, and side-effects are rare. It is, however, *very* dangerous in overdose, when it can result in fatal liver damage. It is very important not to exceed the recommended daily maximum of 4g.

Ibuprofen (brand name Nurofen) is my own choice, but it is not recommended for those who cannot take aspirin, such as asthmatics, nor for people with high blood pressure, kidney problems, or a stomach ulcer. It is important not to exceed the recommended daily maximum of 1.8g, which should not be taken all at once.

Codeine is sold over-the-counter only in the limited form of combinations with other analgesics. It can lead to constipation, and it makes some people feel nauseous, so if you want to avoid this drug, you should check the labels of brand-named combination analgesics and migraine preparations, to be sure it doesn't feature.

Caffeine is also used as an ingredient in analgesics and in some migraine preparations. It is included for its 'mind-lifting' properties, for its shrinking effects on the swollen blood vessels in your head, and because it is thought to enhance the pain-relief. If you are trying to avoid caffeine – or if you want to take a pain-killer and then try to sleep – you should make sure your combination analgesic or migraine preparation does not include caffeine.

TAKING ANALGESICS

Don't exceed the stated dose. This can be dangerous, and it can lead to a range of very unpleasant side-effects. Even a relatively low excess can lead to headaches which are caused by the analgesic itself.

If the pain persists, take a second dose when permitted (usually, after four hours). If that doesn't work, you may need a different pain-killer, or perhaps your pain-killer is not getting through. One of the known effects of migraine is to slow down the action of the gut: gastric stasis occurs. You may need to take the first dose faster, or you may need to add an **anti-sickness drug** (see below). Some migraine drugs contain a combination of analgesics and anti-nauseants, and that might do the trick for you.

2. Anti-sickness drugs

There are several sorts of anti-sickness drugs which can work well for migraine patients in two ways. The drug may stop you feeling nauseous, or stop you vomiting – or both. That will be a great relief to anyone whose experience of migraine centres around the dread of that stage: constantly rushing to vomit, feeling wretched and unhappy, and with a headache made worse by all the constant movement.

The other advantage of two particular anti-nauseant drugs is their effect on the condition called gastric stasis, where nothing is absorbed into your system because the whole digestive process is slowed down during a migraine. These anti-nauseants can make your stomach work effectively again, and so the pain-killer can get to work and relieve the pain. (They are **metoclopromide** and **domperidome**, detailed on the next page.)

Many people who believed they needed stronger pain-killers have found that the use of an anti-nausea drug has transformed their treatment – and the way in which they manage their migraine attacks.

The most usual anti-sickness drugs prescribed for migraine are:

★ Metoclopromide
★ Domperidome
★ Prochlorperazine

★ Buclizine
★ Cyclizine

Metoclopromide is a prescription drug which is available either on its own (Maxolon is a brand name) or as an ingredient in migraine compounds such as Migravess (with aspirin) and Paramax (with paracetamol). It is not recommended for children or young adults, however, and it might make you feel shaky, drowsy, or dizzy.

Domperidome (brand names Evoxin and Motilium) has fewer side-effects, and it is also available as a suppository, which is extremely useful if you have left the treatment a bit late, making your digestion less likely to cope with absorbing the drug's effects.

Prochlorperazine (brand name Stemetil) can also be given in a suppository, but although it is a very powerful anti-nausea drug, this is a less effective choice for keeping the digestion active. It also can cause drowsiness and dizziness.

Buclizine and **cyclizine** are anti-histamines, which can be used to combat nausea in migraine compounds. Migraleve contains buclizine in combination with paracetamol and codeine, while Femigraine contains cyclizine and aspirin.

3. Tranquillisers and sedatives
Diazepam (brand name Valium), **benzodiazepine** (brand name Ativan) and **chlordiazepoxide** (Librium) are sometimes used to help migraineurs relax and lose their tension and anxiety, if those are thought to be triggering the migraine attacks. They can also help to relieve any muscles spasms.

Such drugs can certainly help – but they also carry a

number of potential side-effects which you have probably read about in recent years, including violent mood swings, and the danger of getting hooked. Suddenly stopping the drugs after habituation has occurred can also lead to acute anxiety attacks. However, if your doctor believes that they may help your migraines, the drugs will be prescribed for use only in small doses – in conjunction with pain-killers – to make relaxation and sleep easier. And, since migraine attacks are episodic, you will be taking the drugs infrequently, and so you should avoid the danger of getting hooked. If your doctor recommends them for you and you still feel unhappy, you could discuss the possibility of using them to treat immediate symptoms of anxiety and tension, and make sure you then substitute self-help relaxation techniques instead.

4. Anti-depressants

These are quite commonly used in the treatment of migraine, even when the migraineur is not suffering from depression. (In fact, depression is a common side-effect of migraine: unsurprisingly, when you consider how destructive a force the syndrome can be.) Sometimes it may take a couple of weeks for the effects of these drugs to take hold, and the side-effects in the meantime can include a dry mouth, constipation, drowsiness and blurred vision.

Amitriptyline (brand name Tryptizol) is often used in the treatment of tension headaches, as well as for migraine. It works by blocking the uptake of noradrenaline and serotonin in the bloodstream, and so lifts your mood. Its side-effects can include changes in blood pressure, pulse and heart rhythm, as well as dryness of your mouth, and tremors. Drowsiness can sometimes be avoided by taking the daily dose at night, just before bed.

5. Ergotamine

Brand names such as Cafergot and Migril indicate compounds which include the drug known as ergotamine tartrate. Cafergot also has caffeine in it, and is available in the form of an inhaler as well as tablets, which can be a great advantage for speed of application and effect. Migril also contains an anti-nauseant. Lingraine is a trade name of ergotamine by itself.

Over the years, ergotamine has been a much-prescribed drug for migraine, but it should be used with caution because of its side-effects. It must also be used as intended: it works by constricting swollen blood vessels, and so relieving pain. It should be taken as early as possible in a migraine attack, for maximum effect.

The overuse of ergotamine can have serious side-effects, even for people who take the drug exactly as it is prescribed. If you misunderstand how to use ergotamine, and take too much of it, then the side-effects are even more serious. So you must be sure you know the risks, as well as the possible help.

You must not take more than 6mg to 8mg of ergotamine for any one migraine attack, nor repeat a treatment within any four-day period. And you should not treat more than one migraine attack a week with ergotamine. Even at that recommended level, the side-effects can be unpleasant, including nausea and vomiting, trembling, abdominal pain and muscle cramps, feeling weak, and cold hands and feet. However, those symptoms should wear off after two or three hours.

But if you take ergotamine too frequently – that is, more regularly than every four days – or if you exceed the recommended dose, you may well become addicted to it. You will run the risk of damaged arteries, hallucinations and seizures. More immediately, you will also probably develop much worse headaches – caused by the ergotamine itself. Many people who have fallen into this trap believe that the headaches are migraines, and take more ergotamine to try to cure them: a process which creates almost-constant headaches. And a headache caused by ergotamine will respond only to ergotamine – so taking a pill will relieve the headache, but only for a short time. Sometimes, the dependence becomes so great that patients need to be hospitalised to 'come off' the drug safely.

In healthy people with normal blood pressure, the risk of complications should be rare, but it is still a drug to be considered with great caution. If you are prescribed it, discuss the side-effects carefully with your GP or specialist, and make sure the effects are carefully monitored by both of you.

6. Serotonin-related drugs

The serotonin antagonists are drugs which work by inhibiting the production of neuro-transmitters, especially serotonin (or 5HT, as it's also called). They include **pizotifen** and **methysergide**.

Pizotifen (its brand name is Sanomigran) is a popular migraine preventative, useful for those whose attacks are frequent and long-lasting. It is an anti-histamine as well as an anti-serotonin drug, and its effects can include nausea and drowsiness. One common side-effect with this drug is an increased appetite and related weight gain: many people report putting on a stone or more whilst taking Sanomigran. Some are happy to accept the possibility of weight gain because they are so delighted with the relief from pain they experience.

Pizotifen should be taken every day, and after two weeks your attacks should begin to lessen in frequency and severity; if they do not, you should consult your doctor.

Many doctors believe that **methysergide** (brand name Deseril) should be prescribed only by neurologists, and monitored under strict hospital supervision, because of the severity of its possible side-effects. There is a long list of these, including stomach pains, nausea, vomiting and diarrhoea, mood changes, and restlessness. If it is used, the general rule is to have no more than five months of treatment at a time, followed by at least one month free of the drug.

The newest drug on the migraine market is a serotonin agonist called **sumatriptan**, with the brand name of Imigran. **Sumatriptan** is thought to work by stimulating the serotonin receptors in your brain that control the constriction of blood vessels. It doesn't prevent 5HT from being produced; rather, it affects the way in which it is absorbed. **Sumatriptan** has been shown to relieve or shorten an established migraine attack very effectively: in tests, it has performed better than any other drug.

Its effects can seem miraculous for many people, but it is not without its adverse side-effects. It is also a very expensive drug to prescribe, and some migraineurs find their GPs are reluctant to recommend it for that reason – especially if the doctor's budgets are stretched.

The most usual side-effects of Imigran tablets are nausea, a funny taste in your mouth, dizziness and drowsiness, stiffness in your neck, and a feeling of tightness and pressure anywhere in your body. These are usually mild and not long-lasting. Only one (100mg) tablet should be taken, and if that dose hasn't worked within two or three hours, you may then take an ordinary analgesic, but you must NOT take more Imigran. If your symptoms do go, but then return, you are allowed to take more Imigran – but no more than 300mg in any twenty-four hours.

Imigran is available by injection as well as in tablet form, using a pen-injector. If you want to try it, don't be put off by the thought of injecting yourself – you just hold the pen against your leg, and never even see the needle go in!

The drug is unsuitable for many people (and not prescribed for children, for pregnant women, or for adults over sixty-five), so you should not assume that your problems will end if only you can get your hands on it!

7. Beta-blockers

If you suffer from frequent migraine attacks, and if the attacks are especially severe, you may well want to consider using a prophylactic (preventative) drug.

One group of prophylactic drugs is known as the beta-blockers. These encourage your blood vessels to constrict by slowing your heart rate and so lowering your blood pressure. In fact, this drug was first developed to control angina and high blood pressure and no one knows exactly how it is effective for migraine. The drug works on the beta group of adrenaline receptors in your body, hence its name.

Atenolol and **metoprolol** are highly selective in their action, and have both proved useful in controlling migraine (brand names include Tenormin and Tenoret for **atenolol** and Betolac for **metoprolol**). **Propranolol** (brand names Inderal, Inderetic, and Inderex) may also affect serotonin receptors, and this drug works for many migraine patients.

The side-effects of beta-blockers can include insomnia, lethargy, depression, and nausea. Some people also experience vivid and disquieting dreams. And, of course, because of its effects on the circulatory system, this drug may not be suitable for those with a heart condition. It is not prescribed for asthmatics, or diabetics.

8. Calcium-channel blockers

These drugs work by relaxing the muscles in the walls of your blood vessels, but their effects are disputed. It is thought that the drugs available may be effective because of other actions. They are not presently used in Britain.

9. Other drugs

Clonidine (brand names Dixarit and Catapres) has been widely used for migraine, but more recent research has thrown a great deal of doubt on its effectiveness. Its side-effects can include insomnia and depression, dizziness, constipation, nausea, and skin rashes. It is usually prescribed for women who have migraine and menopausal hot flushes, for it can also relieve those symptoms.

Cyproheptadine is an anti-histamine drug and a serotonin antagonist (see page 159) with the brand name of Periactin. Its side-effects may include drowsiness and headaches, a dry mouth, blurred vision, and weight gain.

Some migraine patients with especially persistent headaches which do not respond to other drug treatments have found relief from a course of monoamine oxidase inhibitor drugs (known, for short, as the **MAO inhibitors**). The drugs work on a group of chemicals which transmit messages between nerve cells in your brain, and they were developed for use in the treatment of depression.

Phenelzine (brand name Nardil) is the one most generally used for migraine. People taking MAO-inhibitor drugs must strictly avoid certain foods like cheese, red wine, chicken livers, and broad beans. They must also avoid certain other drugs (and these include nasal decongestants); the danger of ignoring the list that is issued to patients is very real.

CONCLUSIONS

The range and variety of drugs used to treat migraine is one indication that no one treatment is likely to be completely effective. You should find a drug that enables you to manage your migraine effectively, to reduce or even remove its effects. But a *guaranteed* method of removing the symptoms completely, safely, and effectively has not yet been discovered.

CHAPTER 7

Considering the Alternatives

'I couldn't believe that having my toes wiggled about would help my migraines – but it has!' said one reflexology convert to me. 'I just don't get bad attacks any more.'

'My chiropractor has literally changed my life,' explained another woman. 'She's located the trouble in my neck and treated it, and I've only had one migraine in the last fourteen months.'

'I can't tell you just how wonderful the acupuncture has been. It's like having a life sentence overturned. My migraines have completely disappeared now,' said a young man I interviewed.

In the last ten years there has been a strong revival in interest in 'alternative' – that is, non-drug – treatment for many medical conditions, including migraine.

There are lots of treatments available for migraine outside the drug-centred approach favoured by conventional western medicine. You may find that your local doctor is a member of a medical practice which encourages some of these. Perhaps your local practice even includes treatments such as acupuncture within the services they can offer patients. But most of us will have to seek alternative methods elsewhere, looking to friends and relatives, to chance encounters, or to local community centres and alternative clinics for advice and recommendations about other ways to manage migraine attacks.

Many migraineurs have found help from holistic medicine, and there are certainly lots of advantages in an alternative approach to illness. I have tried quite a few therapies myself, often with good results – although not necessarily permanent ones. And most (though not all) of the people I interviewed who had tried alternative remedies thought they had been helped.

But there may be disadvantages in seeking help – or a cure – from such specialities. So first I want to play devil's advocate, and look at the main disadvantages you should think through.

HAZARD WARNING

1. The cost As long as alternative treatments remain unrecognised or unofficial, their cost is not refunded by any governmental or private insurance system. You might find a medically qualified specialist of some sort who includes an alternative therapy such as acupuncture within part of a whole treatment, but acupuncture alone is seldom covered by the health service, nor can it be claimed back from a private medical insurance company. (Homeopathy can be an exception to this rule; so, in some circumstances, can osteopathic treatment.)

This means that even individual sessions, let alone a course of treatment, can be an expensive matter. For that reason, you may want to consider whether or not you can commit yourself to a course of treatment.

2. Raising the standards Many alternative therapies have a governing body to which properly qualified therapists belong – but some do not. Unless you are very careful about how you select a therapist, you may run the risk of falling into the hands of an unqualified practitioner, who at best won't effect any improvement in your condition, and at worst could do more harm than good.

And in some fields you may be unfortunate enough to encounter a charlatan or a quack, whose only interest is in fleecing you of your money. This happens seldom – but it can still happen. After all, it isn't just the big bad drug companies who are interested in making a profit!

3. Doctor knows best? You should always tell your GP of any plans you have to try an alternative treatment – if only because a proper initial diagnosis would identify any serious medical condition which needs conventional medical attention. And you may find that your GP is unsupportive about the alternative you have chosen, maybe even hostile to the idea.

It's a good idea to listen carefully to all the arguments, but in the end you have to stand your ground, and make your own decisions in the way that seems right to you. If necessary, you can try to find a GP who is more sympathetic to your efforts. They do exist!

Many alternative therapies like to work in harmony with conventional medicine, as a complementary strand of treatment. Others, however, will expect you to abandon your drugs, believing that their treatment will not be effective whilst you are taking them. Understandably, you may well decide not to go along with that suggestion!

4. Is the treatment working? Sometimes it can be difficult to tell if the treatment you receive is really having a permanent effect on your condition. Of course, that's true of conventional drug treatments too. But it is easy to think that an alternative treatment is working in positive ways at first – even if that's not true. The personal, 'holistic' nature of consultation and treatment in alternative medicine can be very soothing and supportive, and so you can feel better for a while just because you and your problems are being attended to with such sympathy. (Psychologists call this the 'attention effect'.) But then, perhaps, the symptoms may recur once more, and only at that stage will you wonder if the treatment has really been effective.

So you will need to decide, in advance, just how long you will allow for the treatment to show results, and you will need to discuss with the therapist what time-span is appropriate. You will also need to be very honest with yourself in judging the effects of the treatment. Again, financial considerations will probably come into play here.

5. The withdrawal effect Many alternative treatments, such as homeopathy, food exclusion diets, and some herbal medicine regimes, will probably induce a 'withdrawal' migraine attack in the first few days, perhaps because you have given up a particular food or drink, or have changed an old ingrained habit. If the treatment is successful, this may be the last migraine attack you will ever suffer, but you should accept that it's on the cards.

167

NATURAL REWARDS

1. The personal touch It makes excellent sense to approach an illness – and especially a complicated syndrome such as migraine – by way of dealing with the whole person, and not just the symptoms. Indeed, it makes such good sense that conventional medical training has begun to concentrate on this long-neglected aspect of healing: the doctor-patient relationship.

A good alternative therapist will take a lot of time to discuss your problems with you, and to devise a programme of treatment that seems best suited to your particular needs.

2. Shopping around In choosing an alternative therapy, you can put to very good use all the research and thought you have expended on your migraine diary, your eating records, and your records of feelings and moods. You may, for example, suspect that your migraine attacks are related to some problem in your neck and shoulders, and you may now know that you have specific muscle pain there at certain points in your migraine 'cycle'. So maybe massage or some form of physiotherapy will help; or treatment from an osteopath or a chiropractor. Or you may decide to try the specialisation of cranial osteopathy, or to look for a craniosacral therapist. All may be worth investigation.

3. The new age feeling Undoubtedly, there are people who find great comfort in the very *idea* of alternative medicine. They approach it in a spirit of positive expectation, and they thoroughly enjoy the process of self-discovery which is often involved in such treatments. Since your attitude to any form of treatment – be it conventional or alternative – is very likely to affect its success or failure, the way you feel about alternative therapy is important. Of course, many people begin with scepticism and end with conviction, but if you begin with a reasonably open mind, you may at least be helping your own treatment along a little.

No treatment can easily withstand an approach from a prospective patient which is based on cynical disbelief, or on that aggressive form of doubt which begins with the conviction that 'this will never work'. If you feel like that about a particular form of treatment, you would do best to avoid it.

CHOOSING A THERAPIST

If you have a personal recommendation, that's good fortune; you can hear all about the good and bad sides of the therapist – and of the treatment – from someone you know.

If that source isn't available to you, you will need to do some research. Ask around; consult the notice boards in your library, and local health food shops. Look in Yellow Pages, and in any local directory of services you can find. If there is a healing centre or alternative treatment clinic in your area, visit it, and talk to the staff about your concerns. Or contact the relevant professional organisations for a list of approved and registered therapists.

It's also an excellent idea to consult the independent bodies – either the Institute of Complementary Medicine, (PO Box 194, London SE16 1QZ), or the British Complementary Medicine Association (The Harold Gillies Unit, St Charles Hospital, Exmoor Street, London WC1). Most properly qualified practitioners of complementary medicine in Britain are registered with one or other of these. (Always enclose a stamped and self-addressed envelope when you are writing for a list of therapists; specify the therapy you are interested in or the problem you want dealt with; and add a couple of loose, first-class stamps to help cover costs.)

If you choose a correctly trained, experienced, and qualified therapist, you stand a good chance of getting the best possible treatment available.

You will then want to meet the therapist for an initial introductory session. The therapist can discuss your problems and come to a conclusion about helping you. You can assess how you will feel about the therapy – and also about the therapist.

The questions you should ask include:

★ Do you think you will be able to help alleviate my migraine attacks?
★ How long will it be before I can expect to notice some improvement in the condition?
★ How long will the course of treatment take?
★ How much will it cost?

A question of empathy
It's important to have a feeling of respect and trust for the person you choose, and you will only be able to begin to assess this when you meet them. Because they try to deal with the whole person and not merely with the symptoms of the illness, many alternative therapies begin (and continue) with searching and personal questions. You won't like those, or find it easy to answer them truthfully, if you don't like the person who's asking them!

SOME THERAPIES TO CONSIDER

I am listing here all the therapies which have been
recommended to me over the years I have spent research-
ing migraine.

Don't take these notes as a substitute for your own
research, enquiries, and interviews with potential therapists. However, reading about what you might expect
from each therapy will give you a good idea of how you
might feel about embarking on such a course of treatment, and what such treatment might involve.

Acupuncture

Although there are different sorts of acupuncture available (the Chinese one, and that developed by conventional
western medicine), the main differences are ones of philosophy, not of treatment.

Western medicine has now adopted acupuncture, and
uses it to treat certain symptoms, but it is not offered as a
cure for any illness.

Chinese acupuncture, on the other hand, aims to treat
your body's underlying imbalances; to restore the proper
relationship between two complementary energy forces –
the Yin and the Yang. Inserting the needles at particular
points in the energy paths throughout the body is thought
to redirect and rechannel its energies in the right ways –
and so to help your body to heal itself. The purpose of
acupuncture is to treat the whole person, not just the
symptoms themselves. Chinese-system acupuncturists
will spend time building up a picture of your general
physical condition.

Opinion differs about the pain involved in acupuncture.
The needles are very fine, and the sensation isn't like a

medical injection. Most people say that they have felt little or no pain at all; others report levels of great discomfort during the treatment. My own experience is somewhere in between those two; I certainly felt the needles go in, and could still feel them whilst they remained in place – but it was more of an ache than real pain.

In the treatment of migraine, you are likely to experience one of two common approaches. The needles are either placed in your ear-lobes, which are thought to represent the body's energy pathways in miniature, or they will be placed in position on your legs, to work on the relevant energy pathways there.

Migraine sufferers often experience relief with acupuncture treatment, but success is by no means universal. It might help to know that, if it is going to work for you, it usually does so within the first few weeks.

One migraineur told me that acupuncture hadn't directly cured her migraines but it had kept her out of 'the foothills of danger' from migraine attacks for a time, and it had restored her energy. *That* gave her the chance to tackle some problems in her life which were triggering migraine. So her migraines have now stopped: directly because of dealing with previously unacknowledged problems, and indirectly because of acupuncture.

The big potential worry about acupuncture these days must probably centre around the possible dangers associated with the needles – such as hepatitis and AIDS. Some practitioners use disposable needles, but of course any qualified and reputable acupuncturist will use only sterilised equipment, and will meticulously follow the Department of Health procedures on sterilisation.

USEFUL ADDRESSES
British Acupuncture Association, 22 Hockley Road, Rayleigh, Essex SS6 8EB.
College of Traditional Chinese Acupuncture, Tao House, Queensway, Leamington Spa, Warwickshire CV31 3LZ.

The Alexander technique

This is a way of examining, and correcting, how your body aligns itself: how you hold yourself, how you walk, sit and move, how your arms and legs relate to your torso, and so on. It is often thought of as a form of exercise, but the lessons do not teach skills which you would usually acquire in an exercise class. You will learn how to realign your body; how to recentre your head on your spine and to support it with the local small muscles rather than with the bigger muscles of your neck. The technique was developed by an actor who needed to rethink the way in which he used (and misused) his voice and his body, and it is still widely used in the acting profession now, sometimes as part of the basic training.

Its relevance to migraine is through the potential trigger of stress and tension – and especially muscular tension. The idea is that once you learn to use your body in a natural and proper way, any problems related to stress can be resolved. And so if you lose, for example, the tension in your neck and shoulders that has been created by awkward body movements and incorrect posture, you will also cut down on any related muscular tension which could trigger a migraine.

There is no possibility of physical discomfort with the Alexander technique; the training given in lessons does not involve any manipulation or stress. But it is not a technique that can be learned quickly, and you will certainly need more than one or two lessons if you are to take seriously the ideas behind the teaching. You would probably need an initial course of perhaps ten forty-minute lessons, and will probably need one or two follow-up courses in later months, to consolidate and extend the progress you make. There are a lot of books about it, too, and you may be able to save session money by consulting them. The one recommended to me by a teacher is *The Alexander Principle* by Dr Wilfred Barlow, published by Arrow.

USEFUL ADDRESSES
The Society of Teachers of the Alexander Technique, 10 London House, 266 Fulham Road, London SW10 9EL.

Aromatherapy
Aromatherapy uses essential oils which are extracted from flowers, herbs, resins and spices for the treatment of various stress-related problems, including migraine. The oils are used in different combinations, and in different ways. They are generally massaged on to your body, but they can also be inhaled, used as a vaporiser or in the bath, or used on compresses. I have heard of therapists who advocate taking the oils by mouth, but that would be an exceptional treatment: most of the oils are far too concentrated for that to be pleasant or safe, and you could damage the mucous lining of your throat and stomach.

Particular oils are used for different remedies: **lovage** oil might be used for a menstrual migraine; **lavender** oil for a stress-related migraine. An aromatherapist will discuss your problems with you, and will blend oils to produce a special mixture just for you. The massage procedure involved in aromatherapy can be immensely soothing and relaxing – and a real help in relieving neck and back tensions.

Everyone I know who's tried 'proper' aromatherapy from a trained therapist (treatment from a beauty therapist can be a disappointment) has had a glorious time, and is convinced that it has helped their migraines in some way. I suspect it's the soothing relaxation and pampering that's the attraction – it certainly is for me! You can learn DIY aromatherapy, but it's a good idea to begin with advice from a qualified practitioner, so you may find it worthwhile to have an initial consultation and then to try out your oils at home.

If your migraines are smell-triggered, you should probably leave having an aromatherapy session until you are in a migraine-free period. Your own specially created oil should be a soothing and delightful smell for you, but you might find a couple of trial oils disturbing, on your way to achieving the right mixture.

USEFUL ADDRESSES
The International Federation of Aromatherapists, Royal Masonic Hospital, Ravenscourt Park, London W6 0TN.

Biochemical tissue salts
You may have seen these on the shelves of your local health food shop, or heard of them in connection with homeopathy. A German homeopathic doctor called Dr Schuessler, developed twelve different salts, corresponding to twelve different minerals, each designed to correct the imbalances in the body chemistry which he believed were responsible for much human illness. The salts are given in minute doses, as are conventional homeopathic

treatments, and it is easy to follow the instructions on the containers.

Since a dose of the appropriate combination of mineral salts is said to restore health, you should soon know if this treatment is doing your migraines any good. You could also try the New Era 'Combination F' tissue salts, which are specially formulated for migraine.

Biofeedback

This is not strictly a therapy, but it is a very successful aid to relaxation, and can be very helpful to migraineurs. All biofeedback techniques work by first giving you information about your body's reactions to certain circumstances, and then by training you to alter those reactions. The advantage is that it shows you when you are relaxed, and it shows you what you did to get there: feedback indeed.

Biofeedback can have very good results in preventing migraine and other headaches which are triggered by tension, and thermal biofeedback is an especially useful preventative because it acts on blood flow.

The bodily processes which can be consciously controlled include blood pressure, heart rate, temperature, and muscle tension. If, for example, muscle tension across your forehead and temples is the problem, you can learn how to control that by having wires attached to the skin of your forehead. The electrical activity generated by contracting muscles can then be amplified, and displayed on a meter or a video screen. Or muscle activity can be turned into a sound that gets louder as the muscles contract, and softer as they relax.

Another device might measure the moisture content of the surface of your skin, or your hand temperature, whilst you learn to concentrate on relaxing, or on making your hands warmer. In this case, two electrodes which measure changes in the surface moisture or the surface temperature of your skin are attached to the palms of your hands or to your fingers, and the machine picks up even the most minute changes. When you feel tense and anxious, you sweat more; when you feel calm and relaxed, you sweat less – and the machine registers those changes.

Thermal biofeedback can help you gain control of your own blood flow. You learn strategies to warm your fingertips, for example, which when put into practice can influence blood flow and prevent a migraine from developing.

Some machines emit a tone which is high when you are anxious, and which falls to a lower note as you relax. A meter or a video display is a better choice for migraineurs who find noise a potential trigger, or for any migraineur who is trying to reduce the severity of an already established attack.

Ask your GP if there is a centre nearby which uses this technique. This could be the psychology department in a university, a healing centre, a stress counselling service, or a pain clinic in a hospital. One firm which manufactures the machines and can train you to use them is Audio Limited, 26 Wendell Road, London W12 9RT.

Chiropractic
A chiropractor treats you by manipulating and adjusting your spine and other joints in your body. If your migraines are associated with back or neck pain, and if you generally feel stiffness and immobility in your shoulders or your back, it may be related to an improper alignment of your spine, and so this therapy could be worth exploring.

The word 'chiropractic' comes from Greek and means

'done by hand', and a chiropractor works on your body by applying pressure on certain bones to encourage them to return to their correct positions. That is done only after a thorough examination, a consultation which includes a full case history, and perhaps also the use of X-rays to complete the diagnosis. Your treatment will also include advice about sleep patterns, posture, and even diet.

Many chiropractic patients report excellent results from their treatments, and complete cures have certainly been effected on some headache and migraine conditions.

USEFUL ADDRESSES
The British Chiropractic Association, 5 First Avenue, Chelmsford, Essex CM1 1RX.
The Institute of Pure Chiropractic, PO Box 126, Oxford OX1 1VF.

Clinical ecology
Doctors who study and treat the field of food allergy and food intolerances are sometimes referred to as clinical ecologists – a term which originated in the United States, where environmental factors such as air pollution were included in the diagnostic process. The term has had bad associations in Britain with cranks, and with bogus diagnostic methods, but nevertheless, it's still a very useful one to describe the ways in which certain substances can cause problems for some people – and how those problems can be dealt with.

There is a difference between food allergy and food intolerance. **Allergy** involves your immune system, and a skin-prick test will produce a positive result; while **intolerance** refers to an adverse reaction to food in which the immune system is not necessarily implicated. Migraine is generally thought to relate only to food intolerances – and, like migraine, food intolerance is a complicated subject which may involve many different factors.

Many migraineurs benefit by avoiding trigger foods, but few find that as a result their migraines clear up altogether. However, clinical ecologists claim that when problem foods are first identified by an **elimination diet** and then avoided, it is common for the migraine attacks to disappear altogether – and for other triggers to be no longer a potential problem.

A clinical ecologist will not ask you to exclude foods from your diet one at a time. Instead, you will be expected to embark on a full elimination diet. The foods will then be reintroduced one at a time, and the ones which cause migraine will thus be identified. The expectation is that more than one food, or food group, will be implicated. (See also pages 66 to 70.)

Diagnostic tests for food intolerance, such as a pulse test, hair analysis, or a cytotoxic test, are not usually thought to be accurate or reliable. Other therapists may suggest the use of rods to test energy fields (metal rods which are held against your body), and it is difficult to judge these. Some reports of such treatments sing the praises of success, and if you have a personal recommendation, it may be worth a try, but it will almost certainly be a costly procedure. (A self-administered elimination diet will be much cheaper – but a lot more trouble for you.)

However, it may be worth trying if your migraines are causing you great and frequent distress, especially if you have other symptoms of allergy or intolerance as well. But for those of us whose migraines have a different or broken pattern, it would be hard to judge the success of an elimination diet within a short period of time – and you might want to try a therapy which invades less of your life.

A list of allergy clinics within the NHS is available – but only to GPs and not to the general public – from The British Society and Clinical Immunology Secretariat, 55 New Cavendish Street, London W1M 7RE. And for a list of registered nutritionists, apply to ICM (see page 169).

USEFUL ADDRESSES
Action Against Allergy, 24–26 High Street, Hampton Hill, Middlesex TW12 1PD.

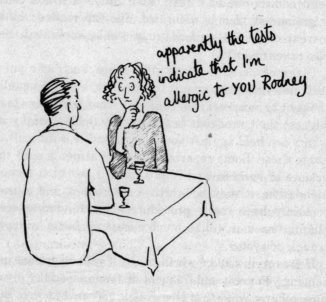

apparently the tests indicate that I'm allergic to YOU Rodney

The British Society for Allergy and Environmental Medicine, 66 Station Road, Fulbourn, Cambridge CB1 5ES.

Craniosacral therapy

The difference between this therapy and cranial osteopathy (see under **osteopathy**) is very like that between medical and traditional Chinese acupuncture: it is more a difference of philosophy than of technique. Both use their hands to 'listen' to your body, but craniosacral therapists will always have a pronounced 'holistic' approach to their work, and will often concentrate on soft tissue as well as bone structures. The touch and manipulation involved are usually very gentle – even rather subtle. Feelings of congestion and tension in your skull and spine can often be relieved by this treatment, and sometimes just one session can bring excellent results.

USEFUL ADDRESSES
The Craniosacral Therapy Association, 3 Sandgrove Cottages, Horsley, Nailsworth, Gloucestershire GL6 0PS.

Herbal medicine

Herbs have been used throughout history, and in almost every culture, for medical treatments. Many conventional drugs have their origin in herbal extracts, and many famous systems – such as Chinese medicine and the Indian Ayurvedic medicine – are based on herbal treatments. For migraine, the most famous self-help herbal remedy is **feverfew** (see pages 140 to 143) but other treatments are available through practitioners such as

181

medical herbalists, whilst many alternative treatments involve peripheral use of herbs – such as aromatherapy, and the Hawaiian Na Pua Olohe body massage.

The treatments will vary according to the practitioner, the exact branch of herbal medicine which is being used, and your particular symptoms. It may include tinctures, tablets or dried herbs, as well as relaxation therapy. Your diagnosis will not be based solely on your symptoms, however; it will include other aspects of your mental and bodily well-being.

The results of medical herbalist treatment for migraine have been varied, but some sorts of migraine (hormonally related, for example) have shown very good results. It may, however, take quite a long time to achieve these in full, perhaps a year or more.

USEFUL ADDRESSES
National Institute of Medical Herbalists, 9 Palace Gate, Exeter, EX1 1JA.

For a list of registered practitioners of Chinese medicine, contact ICM (see page 169).

Homeopathy
This can be available on the NHS. There are GPs who practise it, five hospitals in Britain which specialise in homeopathic treatments, and many chemists which stock homeopathic treatments. Many practising homeopaths also have medical qualifications.

Homeopathy works on the idea of 'like cures like', and so the treatment will involve minute doses of substances such as herbal extracts, salts, and minerals. For example, if a substance for treating migraine were given to normal people, it would produce the symptoms of migraine. Homeopathy, it is believed, stimulates your body into curing itself of the problem.

Self help is possible with homeopathy – you can buy the pills, and read books about diagnosis and treatment – but this is not recommended for migraine. You should consult a practitioner who will prescribe for you as an individual. A homeopath will not merely treat your symptoms, but will spend a great deal of time building up a picture of your total health and background.

Homeopathy can be very helpful for hormonally related or stress-related migraine. It may be that your migraine will respond almost immediately to a homeopathic course of treatment, but sometimes the condition gets worse before it improves, and you would need to be prepared for that possibility.

One woman I talked to has been successfully treated for both psoriasis and migraine, and has not had an attack for eighteen months. Initially she found it difficult to give up coffee and peppermints (their elimination was an essential part of her treatment), and was also anxious about the possible results of abandoning her regular medications. 'I can't even take anything for a bad cold,' she explained, 'but sometimes a bit of adjustment in the timing of taking my regular homeopathic remedies can help there. And I'm so delighted to be migraine-free that the price seems insignificant.'

Useful Addresses
The Faculty of Homoeopathy, Royal London Homoeopathic Hospital, Great Ormond Street, London WC1N 3HR.
British Homoeopathic Association, 27a Devonshire Street, London W1N 1RJ.

Hypnotherapy

This is a very useful relaxation procedure to learn. Self-hypnosis can be taught in one or two sessions, and can be put into practice almost anywhere, to relieve stress and tension, and to increase your self-awareness and well-being. Hypnosis is not a cure for migraine; it's just one way of dealing with stress which may suit you. I have found it a great help, especially because I was taught the techniques of self-hypnosis, which I regularly use to deal with stress.

Some people are frightened by the idea of being hypnotised, believing that in some way they will be 'made' to do things against their will – but the truth is very different. Hypnosis produces, and then uses, a particular state of mind: a different sort of awareness, which is accompanied by a deep physical relaxation. At each stage of relaxation in the 'trance', you can choose to sink deeper into relaxation, to stay where you are, or to pull back out. Some people are certainly more suggestible than others, but the techniques has been used successfully on migraine, because of the relaxed state which it induces.

The strategies you learn in hypnosis enable you to find different ways of dealing with the trials of daily life, a difficult or demanding job or family, and so on. If you have trouble relaxing, or if you allow things to wind you up, then learning the techniques of self-hypnosis would help a lot. The visualisation practice, in particular, is a great strength for many people. Of course, you don't have to choose this method of relaxation – there are other techniques which use the same visualisation tools, and the same sort of levels of awareness.

You must make sure you visit a hypnotist who is

properly qualified, and a member of one of the relevant organisations.

The National Council of Psychotherapists and Hypnotherapy Register, 46 Oxhey Road, Watford WD1 4QQ.

Massage
Massage has been used as a therapy for illness for thousands of years, and it is a delightfully sensuous way to ease aches and pains, to release stiffness and tension associated with migraine headaches, and to soothe tensions. It helps with blood pressure problems, stimulates your blood flow and your lymphatic system, deals with localised problems such as neck pain or stiffness of your lower back, and reduces joint swelling and pain.

You don't have to be ill to have a massage, but it can certainly help migraine. A specific area massage, such as neck, shoulders and upper back, can relieve or remove a migraine headache, or cope with the post-drome period's aches and pains, and sensitivities. You can learn to massage bits of your own body, but you would have to be a contortionist to reach that critical part for many migraineurs: the upper back and spine. Some migraineurs have learned some basic massage techniques, and have exchange sessions with their partners or with other migraineurs ('you massage my back today and I'll do yours next week . . .'). Some people learn to treat their acupressure points (see pages 124 to 136), or ask friends or partners to do that for them during a migraine attack.

Of all the alternative therapies, this is my own favourite, and a life-saver when stress levels seem to be spiralling out of control. I save up for a massage treatment every six weeks or so – and when I can't afford one, my body begins to complain!

Many women prefer to find a female masseur, and that's very easy these days. Most healing centres will have a list of both male and female practitioners, and most gyms and clubs will also be able to help. You should only use a qualified person, preferably one registered with ICM (see page 169).

Meditation

This is another useful form of relaxation therapy which has been very beneficial to many whose migraines are stress- and tension-related. (And, as one person cheerfully pointed out, 'once you've learned it, it's free!')

Meditation can incorporate many diffferent theories and processes, and blends well with your own style of approaching things. You don't have to sit cross-legged and say 'Om' if that makes you feel uncomfortable or foolish, and you don't have to contemplate a flower, or your navel, if you'd rather not. It's important to choose a school of thought which appeals to you, so you need to decide whether a movement-based technique, or a mind-based one, is likely to meet your needs.

The Alexander technique and other forms of movement therapy such as t'ai chi and yoga, hypnotherapy, and other forms of mind therapy such as counselling, can all incorporate or lead to ways of reaching a meditative state. You can concentrate on physical or mental meditations; you can learn to control bodily processes such as your heart rate or your blood pressure through meditation. It can be extremely useful as a technique for dealing with the changed life-style implications of migraine, and it can give you renewed enthusiasm and energy.

If you want to try do-it-yourself meditation, it will probably be easiest to begin with a mental programme, but it will certainly help to begin with some instruction. Many health centres and local authorities run meditation classes, so check with your doctor or your local library for details, or contact an adult education centre.

Naturopathy

A naturopath believes that your body's illness is a sign of its efforts to regain health, and so the symptoms your body produces are encouraged, rather than suppressed. For this reason, and because of the dietary restrictions imposed by a naturopathic regime, migraineurs who put themselves in the hands of a naturopath can expect an initial 'withdrawal' migraine attack – and you must be prepared for that to occur.

However off-putting that may sound, many aspects of naturopathic treatment fit into the known patterns of migraine attack, and naturopathy is certainly worth considering. The basic causes of illness which a naturopath will look at fall into three groups: chemical imbalances; mechanical problems of functioninng within the nervous systems and the muscular and skeletal systems; and the psychological factor. Treatment can include a largely raw-food diet; hydrotherapy; remedial exercises or osteopathic treatment; and relaxation techniques. (It can also include fasting, so be prepared to reject that alternative if you feel it wouldn't be wise for you.)

USEFUL ADDRESSES
The British College of Osteopathy and Naturopathy, 6 Netherhall Gardens, London NW3 5RR.

Osteopathy

The difference between this therapy and its close relative, chiropractic therapy, can be difficult to distinguish if you are not 'in the know'. Basically, chiropractors work by exerting pressure on your bones, and its felt effects are usually reasonably gentle. An osteopath, however, will manipulate your bones and muscles to correct the ways in which they are aligned, and to free particular joints.

Osteopaths are trained to detect even the most minute problems in your spinal structure, and the consultation will probably include a note of your posture and the way you sit, stand, and move.

The manipulation *can* seem rather alarming. It's not necessarily painful, but you can certainly feel what's happening, and you may well be twisted, pushed, and pulled into odd positions, and your joints stretched, or put under pressure. You will probably hear – and feel – a cracking noise as the vertebrae in your spine are repositioned, and you may feel a bit stiff and sore afterwards.

For those whose migraines are caused by stiffness or misalignment in neck, shoulders and back, however, the slight unpleasantness is well compensated by a relief from deep-seated pain. The treatment may include various applications of heat as well, and it is said to correct blood flow problems as well as muscular spasm.

Sometimes one or two treatments are all that are required, perhaps with a follow-up if the problems reappear.

One specific osteopathic treatment for migraine which receives excellent reports is **cranial osteopathy**. This is a technique which involves very gentle pressure on the bones of the skull, and which corrects misalignment of the 'plate-like' joins. Again, an osteopath trained in this specialisation will look for minute areas of difficulty, and sometimes the effects of this almost imperceptible therapy can be astounding. (See also page 181.)

(See also page 181.)

USEFUL ADDRESSES
The British College of Osteopathy and Naturopathy (see under **Naturopathy**).
British Osteopathic Association, 8–10 Boston Place, London NW1 6HQ.

Reflexology

Sometimes also called **zone therapy**, this is a version of acupressure which concentrates on the feet, so the treatment consists of a gentle but searching massage which deals with each separate area of your feet. For many people, the very idea of having their feet massaged is so glorious that the philosophy behind the therapy gets less attention, but it is an interesting relative of acupressure with the same basic ideas about energy fields – in this case, related to specific zones in the feet and ankles which correspond to specific areas of your body. So the sinus area can be stimulated by pressure to the pads of your toes; the sciatic nerve by pressure to an area of your heel, and so on.

Problem areas often respond by feeling tender or painful under pressure, so reflexology is used as a diagnostic treatment as well as a therapy. Since it can help stress-related problems, and is often recommended for menstrual and menopausal problems as well as for migraine and general headaches, it is probably not surprising that many migraineurs report beneficial effects from this treatment, and try to save up for a treatment every month or two.

USEFUL ADDRESSES
International Institute of Reflexology, PO Box 34, Harlow, Essex.

Shiatsu massage

An easy way to describe this massage/physiotherapy is to refer to it as the Japanese version of acupressure. The word means 'finger pressure' in Japanese, and a philosophy similar to that involved in acupuncture, involving energy fields and energy points around your body, lies behind the treatment.

It is done while you are wearing some sort of loose clothing – a track suit, say – and the pressure will be applied in a very different way from the sort of conventional massage that has been developed in other therapies in the western world. The masseur may use her fingers or just her thumbs, maybe her hands or elbows, perhaps even knees or feet, to apply different sorts of pressure to various parts of your body, to rebalance its energy, and to release blockages in energy paths. Sometimes the pressure on particular points can be painful, but the whole experience is generally relaxing, and often invigorating too. Some aspects work well as self-help treatment at home, between sessions.

Shiatsu massage is often found to relieve migraine and other headaches, and is one of the forms of massage which is recommended for period pains. It is also very effective when it is combined with some form of relaxation therapy.

USEFUL ADDRESSES
Shiatsu Society, 19 Langside Park, Kilbarchan, Renfrewshire PA10 2EP.

Spiritual healing

The idea of spiritual healing, and of people who are able to heal others by the laying on of hands, is at least as old as recorded history. It involves the belief that some people can 'tap into' an energy force which can be channelled from one person to another: in this case, from the healer to the person who is ill. Usually this involves a physical connection (hence the 'laying on of hands'), but sometimes the healing can be effected at a distance, by positive thought processes. If you are a conventionally minded person, this probably sounds about as extreme – and loopy – an alternative therapy as possible, yet healers are allowed to work within some NHS hospitals in Britain, and some GPs are learning to use this process, too. It shouldn't be dismissed without thought.

It is difficult to understand how such a process might work – but that it *does* work, in some cases and for some people, cannot be denied. Sceptics will claim that some other process is at work – such as spontaneous remission, self-persuasion, or perhaps the attention effect – but trials in the States have apparently shown better-than-placebo results for therapeutic touch. Patients who have found this useful report deep feelings of relaxation and loss of tension, as well as the cessation of symptoms.

Spiritual healers don't claim that this therapy always works, and it doesn't. But I have certainly heard reports of cures for migraine described with conviction, and it may be that this therapy would be a helpful one for you to consider.

USEFUL ADDRESSES
National Federation of Spiritual Healing, Old Manor Farm Studio, Church Street, Sunbury on Thames, Middlesex TW16 6RG.

Yoga

Yoga isn't just a therapy; it's a spiritual philosophy which involves physical therapy, and which is thought to benefit your body, mind, and spirit in harmonious combination. Migraineurs who choose yoga as their relaxation therapy often report excellent results, probably through a reduction in stress and tension levels, and perhaps also through the gentle physical stretching and breathing exercises which yoga classes involve.

You don't necessarily have to take the philosophy on board to enjoy yoga, or to benefit from it. It's an excellent form of exercise to choose because of its gentle, unstressful nature. Classes are often run as part of adult education schemes, and are not usually expensive. You would need to plan on at least a term of once-a-week classes to start with; the techniques take time to learn, and the stress-reduction will take time to begin to work.

USEFUL ADDRESSES
British Wheel of Yoga, 80 Leckhampton Road, Cheltenham, Gloucestershire.

CHAPTER 8

The Search Continues

As you will have gathered by now, finding a cure for migraine is a tricky business. Most people can learn to manage their migraines and make the attacks less severe, and many people have managed to rid themselves of migraine – but that's not the same as identifying a cure, since migraine is a complicated syndrome with many potential causes. But there are some very hopeful developments, and some really positive signs for the future.

INTEREST IN MIGRAINE

One of the most cheering developments is the sheer level of attention that migraine now receives. The general public has become more aware of the issues involved in migraine, and this in turn has stimulated more understanding amongst researchers and GPs.

Research on individual trigger factors has produced some useful results, although lots more work needs to be done. And, while the development of individual drugs to relieve or to prevent the symptoms of migraine has recently produced some very effective treatments, a drug is not necessarily the best solution. Many sufferers would avoid drugs if they could find a reliable and effective alternative. Yet at present, alternative and holistic medicine provide no more complete an answer than conventional medicine does.

Work continues in laboratories and clinics around the world. Scientists are studying blood vessels, and measuring cerebral blood flow. It is now possible to measure the brain's metabolism, and that means it may soon be possible to say exactly which parts of the brain are affected during a migraine attack. Chemical reactions in the human nervous system are being studied to isolate the exact variations in supply and production which occur in your body. The search for a diagnostic test for migraine continues, too, with new results soon expected from work with EEGs.

Other studies are concentrating on the psychological basis of migraine, and on the various physical factors which can affect your mind and your body. And in the last year, the British Association for the Study of Headache (known as BASH) was formed. This has a scientific and educational role, and intends actively to promote the study of headache. There's certainly good reason to hope that migraine will be defeated, some time in the near future.

Doing something about your own migraines needs a sustained effort from you, and from other support systems. There are a number of possible ways in which you could extend your own understanding of migraine, receive specialised support and guidance – *and* do something towards further research which might help other people, as well as yourself, in the future.

The Migraine Clinics

There are specialised migraine and general headache clinics all over the world. Some are self-contained units, while others are linked to the neurological departments of hospitals. Some excellent research results have come from the work carried out at migraine clinics, and their continued development and expansion can do nothing but good.

If you are referred to a migraine clinic, you will be seen by doctors with a special interest in migraine and an up-to-date knowledge of treatment procedures and techniques. Many doctors working in migraine clinics are themselves migraine sufferers, so their understanding is especially comprehensive!

One of the great advantages for both the migraineur and the doctor is that migraine clinics will see people without referrals when they are experiencing an acute attack. This means that the best treatment will be provided immediately. You will be given drugs if that's appropriate, and then left in a dark and quiet room to sleep off the worst of the migraine. And research that includes experience of the attack itself has been enormously important, because understanding this vital, central period is critical. (It is, after all, the piece of the puzzle which is often missing from your GP's experience and understanding of migraine.)

If you think that your medical treatment for migraine has not been as successful as you'd wish, or if you want to take advantage of a particular clinic's specialisations (for example, in the treatment of hormonally related migraine), you can ask your GP to refer you to a particular place. You may have to wait several months for an appointment, but remember that you can receive treatment without referral during an acute attack, if things get too bad in the meantime.

Some migraine clinics specialise in research into a particular alternative treatment, such as acupuncture. And many clinics regularly ask for volunteers to help with specific research.

The British Migraine Association

This organisation has three main aims: to encourage and support migraine research; to be a sort of 'clearing-house' between the medical and scientific community and ordinary migraineurs for information about migraine drugs and treatments; and to provide encouragement, support, and understanding for migraineurs. Members receive twice-yearly newsletters and special leaflets filled with information, suggestions, reminders, and practical advice. It is a life-line of comfort and positive support for many people. (See page 198 for address details.)

Support and Self-Help Groups

If you have one of these already established in your area, you are very lucky! Join it immediately, and attend the group meetings – for nothing is more helpful than to meet other migraineurs, to discuss triggers and treatments, and to learn about the ways in which others manage their attacks.

If there is not a group near you, you should seriously consider starting one up. There are often advertisements in the British Migraine Association newsletter asking for contacts in local areas, and you could place one yourself. The Association has also produced a leaflet on the subject, to help you get started.

The Leicester Migraine Self-Help Group are unique, as far as I (and they) know, in having an enormously practical and positive approach to tackling migraine. If you are a migraineur living in or near Leicester, you're in luck! Contact them through the secretary: tel: (0533) 414309.

The Migraine Trust

This London-based organisation has been established for more than twenty-five years, and was founded to promote medical research into migraine. It funds research in hospitals and universities; funds the establishment of new migraine clinics, and helps support some of the existing clinics; organises and runs the bi-annual International Migraine Symposium, where leading migraine experts from around the world meet to exchange information and ideas about research ideas. It also provides an information service to the general public.

LOOKING A-HEAD

Its most recent initiative is to create a new advisory committee which will act as a clearing-house to exchange information from migraine clinics about the latest developments in patient care. This will ensure that comprehensive information is easily available to both GPs and patients. It is also supporting the establishment of a new range of migraine clinics: the aim is at least one migraine clinic in each regional health authority area.

A Migraine Trust patient support group now also exists in London, where migraineurs can meet to share experiences, have access to the latest information, and help raise funds for future research. For further details, contact the address on page 198.

Useful Addresses
in Britain

The British Migraine Association,
178a High Road,
Byfleet, West Byfleet,
Surrey KT14 7ED.
Tel: (0932) 352468.

The Migraine Trust,
45 Great Ormond Street,
London WC1N 3HZ.
Tel: (071) 278 2676.

THE MIGRAINE CLINICS

(Emergency treatment is available at the start of a
migraine attack; otherwise you will need a referral from
your GP.)

London

The City of London Migraine Clinic,
22 Charterhouse Square,
London EC1M 6DX.
Tel: (071) 251 3322.

The Princess Margaret Migraine Clinic,
Charing Cross Hospital,
Fulham Palace Road,
London W6 8RF.
Tel: (081) 846 1252.

Britain

The Migraine Clinic,
Royal Victoria Hospital,
Grosvenor Road,
Belfast BT12 6BA.
Tel: (0232) 240503.

The Migraine Clinic,
Queen Elizabeth Hospital,
University Department of Neurology,
Edgbaston,
Birmingham B15 2TH.
Tel: (021) 627 2080.

The Migraine Clinic,
Royal Preston Hospital,
Sharoe Green Lane,
Preston PR2 4HT.
Tel: (0772) 710423.

The Migraine Clinic,
Oldchurch Hospital,
Romford, Essex
Tel: (0708) 345533.

The Migraine Clinic,
Bootham Park Hospital,
Bootham,
York YO3 7BY.
Tel: (0904) 610777.

The neurological departments of many hospitals will also
see migraine patients. Your GP will know if any near you
offer that service, and you will in any case need a referral
from your GP.

International
Migraine Associations

Australia: Migraine Society of Australia, PO Box 2504, Kent Town Centre, South Australia 5071.

Canada: The Migraine Foundation, 120 Carlton Street, Ste 210, Toronto, Ontario.

Denmark: Migraenikerforbundet, Post Box 1232, 5100 Odense C.

India: Dr A.N. Pande, 113/57 Swaroop Nagar, Kanpur 208002.

Netherlands: Nederlandse Vereniging, Van Migraine-patienten Postbus 50, 7037 ZG Beek, GE.

New Zealand: Executive Director, New Zealand Neurological Fund, PO Box 68402, Auckland 1.

Sweden: Swedish Migraine Association, Banergarten 55, 11553 Stockholm.

USA: American Pain Society, 340 Kingsland Street, Nutley, New Jersey 07110.
National Migraine Foundation, 5252 North Western

Avenue, Chicago, Illinois 60625.

Rocky Mountain Headache Association, 1155 East 18th Avenue, Denver, Colorado 80218.

Further Reading

RELATED TOPICS

The Alexander Principle, Dr Wilfred Barlow (Arrow, 1984)

The British Medical Association Guide to Medicine and Drugs (Dorling Kindersley, 1991)

E for Additives, Maurice Hanssen and Jill Marsden (Thorsons, 1984)

Food Allergy and Intolerance, Dr Jonathan Brostoff and Linda Gamlin (Bloomsbury, revised 1992)

Food Combining for Health; a new look at the Hay system, Doris Grant and Jean Joice (Thorsons, 1991)

Stress and Relaxation, Jane Madders (Macdonald, 1981)

Superfoods, Michael van Straten and Barbara Griggs (Dorling Kindersley, 1990)

MIGRAINE BOOKS

Migraine, Oliver Sacks (Picador, revised edition 1993)

The Migraine Handbook, Jenny Lewis with The Migraine Association (Vermilion, 1993)

The Migraine Revolution, Dr John Mansfield (Thorsons, 1986)

Migraine Special Diet Cookbook, Cecilia Norman (Thorsons, 1990)

Migraine: a spectrum of ideas, ed. J. Merton Sandler and Geralyn Collins (Oxford University Press, 1990)

Understanding Headaches and Migraines, Dr J.N. Blau (*Which?* Consumer Guides, 1991)

Understanding Migraine, Dr Marcia Wilkinson and Dr Anne MacGregor (Family Doctor Publications, 1993)

Index

More Non-Fiction from Headline:

Sexual Awareness

Enhancing Sexual Pleasure

Barry and Emily McCarthy

ILLUSTRATED   NEW UNEXPURGATED EDITION

This book is written to show individuals and couples how to enhance their sexual pleasure. It is focused on feelings and fulfilment, and emphasizes a joyful expression of sexuality and intimacy.

The path to a new awareness includes chapters on:
The Pleasure of Touching
Self-Exploration
Increasing Arousal For Women
Becoming Orgasmic
Learning Control
Overcoming Inhibition

With the current emphasis on the importance of just one sexual partner, this is a timely publication designed to show you just how to make the most of that relationship, and how to build a new sexual partnership.

NON-FICTION/REFERENCE   0 7472 3561 9

JUST THE ONE

THE WIVES AND TIMES OF
JEFFREY BERNARD

G R A H A M   L O R D

'One of the most thoroughly researched biographical enquiries I have read. It's all here, booze, women, Norman Balon, horses, "No-knickers Joyce", booze, and finally fame of a sort a writer rarely achieves in his lifetime' Patrick Marnham, *The Oldie*

Jeffrey Bernard, the legendary Soho journalist and boozer who has been popping down to the pub for 'just the one' for forty years is the most unlikely hero of our times.

What other bottle-of-vodka-and-fifty-fags-a-day hack has also been a gigolo, navvy, fairground boxer, miner, stagehand, film editor and actor? Who else has been married four times, seduced 500 lovers (including several renowned actresses) – and also written a famous column for the *Spectator*, his 'suicide note in weekly instalments'? In the astonishingly successful stage play, *Jeffrey Bernard is Unwell*, his rackety life has been portrayed by Peter O'Toole, Tom Conti, James Bolam and Dennis Waterman.

Graham Lord – who has known Bernard well for many years – has written a biography that is fun, devastatingly frank and critical, yet unexpectedly touching. Jeffrey Bernard is indeed unique – just the one.

'I wanted it to be longer. I read it from cover to cover in one sitting and laughed out loud and often' Paul Pickering, *Sunday Times*

'A gripping and unsentimental biography...an astonishing achievement' Irma Kurtz, *Sunday Express*

NON-FICTION/BIOGRAPHY   0 7472 4286 0

Headline Health Kicks

Positive and practical advice to relieve persistent health problems.
Titles available include:

THE PRIME OF YOUR LIFE
Self help during menopause   Pamela Armstrong   £5.99   ☐

STOP COUNTING SHEEP
Self help for insomnia sufferers   Dr Paul Clayton   £5.99   ☐

AM I A MONSTER, OR IS THIS PMS?
Self help for PMS sufferers   Louise Roddon   £5.99   ☐

GET UP AND GO!
Self help for fatigue sufferers   Anne Woodham   £5.99   ☐

You can kick that problem!

All Headline books are available at your local bookshop or newsagent, or can be ordered direct from the publisher. Just tick the titles you want and fill in the form below. Prices and availability subject to change without notice.

Headline Book Publishing Ltd, Cash Sales Department, Bookpoint, 39 Milton Park, Abingdon, OXON, OX14 4TD, UK. If you have a credit card you may order by telephone – 0235 831700.

Please enclose a cheque or postal order made payable to Bookpoint Ltd to the value of the cover price and allow the following for postage and packing:

UK & BFPO: £1.00 for the first book, 50p for the second book and 30p for each additional book ordered up to a maximum charge of £3.00.

OVERSEAS & EIRE: £2.00 for the first book, £1.00 for the second book and 50p for each additional book.

Name..

Address..

....

....

If you would prefer to pay by credit card, please complete:
Please debit my Visa/Access/Diner's Card/American Express (delete as applicable) card no:

☐☐☐☐☐☐☐☐☐☐☐☐☐☐☐☐☐☐☐

Signature...   Expiry date...................